STOMACH ULCER DIET GUIDE

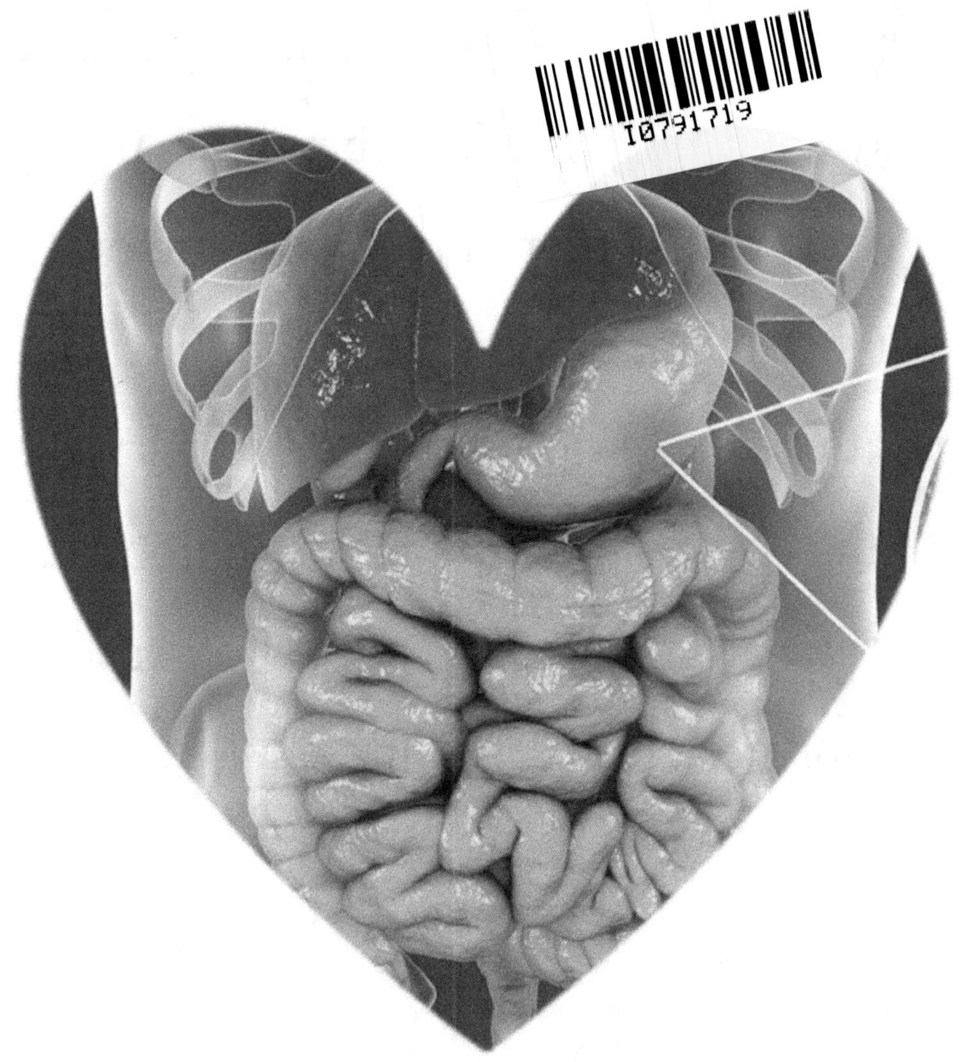

DEBORAH D. CLEARY

Disclaimer

This book's characters, events, and circumstances are entirely fictional. Any similarity to natural persons, living or deceased, or actual events is coincidental.

The opinions expressed by the characters in this work do not necessarily reflect those of the author. The author does not endorse specific beliefs, ideologies, or actions in the narrative.

This book is a work of fiction created for entertainment purposes only. The author makes no guarantees or warranties regarding the accuracy or completeness of the contents, explicitly disclaiming all warranties, including fitness for a particular purpose.

Readers are encouraged to form opinions and judgments about the content and seek professional advice if necessary. The author is not responsible for any direct, indirect, consequential, or incidental damages arising from the use of information provided in this book.

About the Author

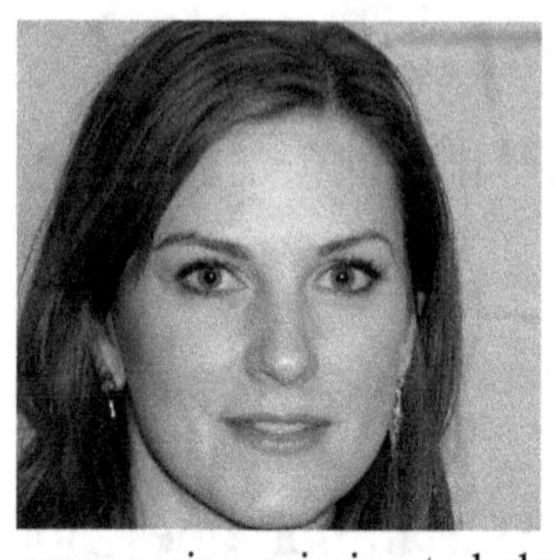

Hello! I'm Deborah Cleary, a nutritionist and medical doctor dedicated to enhancing the health and well-being of my patients through holistic and practical approaches. With a deep understanding of the intricate connections between nutrition, hormones, and overall health, I have made it my unwavering mission to help individuals achieve optimal wellness.

As a mother of three beautiful children, I know firsthand the importance of family and the challenges of maintaining a balanced and healthy lifestyle in a busy household. My experiences have not only deepened my commitment to helping others navigate their health journeys but also made me more empathetic and understanding, providing practical advice and easy-to-follow guidance.

My passion for making people happy and healthy has remained a driving force throughout my professional journey. By combining my medical expertise with my nutritional knowledge, I strive to offer comprehensive, science-based solutions that empower my readers and patients to take control of their health. My approach goes beyond treating symptoms, focusing instead on fostering lasting, positive changes through sustainable lifestyle choices.

In this book, I share the insights and practices I have learned and refined over years of study and practice. My goal is to provide you with accessible, delicious recipes and practical meal plans that support hormonal balance and overall well-being. With a warm, family-centered approach, I want to clarify that my primary aim is to help you live a healthier, happier life.

Join me on a journey to better health and discover how the right foods and lifestyle choices can profoundly affect your life.

Table of Contents

CHAPTER FOUR: Cooking Techniques for Ulcer-Friendly Meals 67

CHAPTER FIVE: Medications and Natural Remedies   81

CHAPTER SIX: Recipes for Ulcer Patients   95

INTRODUCTION

You're at the dinner table, surrounded by your favorite dishes, but something has changed. What was once a joyous occasion is now fraught with anxiety. You bite, and the familiar searing sensation sets in before you know it. It's aggravating, even frightening, and you start to worry if you'll ever enjoy eating without fear again.

If this resonates with you, please know that you are not alone. Stomach ulcers can make eating seem like a battle, turning something as easy as a meal into a cause of anxiety. But this book exists to help you regain control of your health, one bite at a time.

Welcome to the **Stomach Ulcer Diet Guide**, a caring companion created with your healing in mind. I realize how difficult it can be—the ambiguity, the irritation, the continual worry about what you should and shouldn't eat. Perhaps you've tried various diets or drugs, and nothing seems to provide long-term comfort. It's easy to become discouraged, but I'm here to assure you that there is hope.

This guide is more than rules and restrictions; it provides the skills to fuel your body while aiding your healing process. Yes, we'll look at the science behind stomach ulcers and how they're affected by the food you eat, but we'll also talk about comfort—finding joy in meals again, feeling empowered to make pain-free choices, and, most importantly, self-care.

It's expected to be concerned, even terrified, about your health. Those feelings are valid. But through this book, I hope to provide you with encouragement and confidence as we embark on this adventure together. We'll discuss practical guidance, calming foods, and tactics that make sense for your lifestyle. I want you to feel secure, not overwhelmed, knowing that making tiny, meaningful changes can provide significant relief.

I understand that this journey may seem frightening, but I encourage you to approach it with curiosity and calm. Healing does not happen overnight, and that is okay. It's a process, and this book will lead you through each stage. You're not simply managing your symptoms; you're gaining control of your health, which is something to be proud of.

So, while turning these pages, remember you're in a safe environment. This handbook was produced with empathy, understanding, and the desire for a better, healthier future for you. Take your time, listen to your body, and believe healing is achievable. I promise you'll discover more than just guidance here—a sense of relief and a reminder that you deserve to feel good.

Let us start on the path to recovering your health, one meal at a time. You've got this, and I'll be with you every step of the way.

Let's Get Started!!!

CHAPTER ONE: Understanding Stomach Ulcers

A stomach ulcer, also called a gastric ulcer, is a lesion that forms on the stomach's lining. It is a form of peptic ulcer, a more extensive term that covers ulcers in the upper part of the small intestine (duodenal ulcers) and, less commonly, the esophagus. These ulcers arise when the stomach's protective mucus layer, which protects the stomach lining from acidic digestive juices, is destroyed or impaired. When this happens, the stomach's powerful acids destroy the tissue, producing an open sore.

Types of Stomach Ulcers

1. Gastric Ulcer.

Gastric ulcers are peptic ulcers that occur on the stomach's inner lining. This happens when the protective mucus layer that protects the stomach lining from digestive acids is damaged, allowing the acid to erode the stomach lining and form an open sore. Gastric ulcers are more likely to cause pain after eating since the stomach releases acid to break down food. This form of ulcer can be caused by H. pylori infection, long-term use of NSAIDs, or other factors such as smoking and heavy alcohol intake.

2. Duodenal Ulcer.

A duodenal ulcer originates in the duodenum, the first section of the small intestine, just beyond the stomach. Unlike gastric ulcers, pain from duodenal ulcers typically begins a few hours after eating or when the stomach is empty at night. The exact reasons for stomach ulcers, such as H. pylori infection and NSAID use, often cause duodenal ulcers. However, they are more common than stomach ulcers and are frequently associated with high acid levels.

3. Esophageal ulcer

An esophageal ulcer forms in the esophagus, transporting food from the mouth to the stomach. These ulcers are commonly caused by gastroesophageal reflux disease (GERD), which occurs when stomach acid rushes back into the esophagus, irritating the lining. Over time, acid reflux can damage the esophagus and cause ulcers. Other causes include heavy alcohol consumption, smoking, or swallowing caustic substances. Esophageal ulcers can cause throat pain, heartburn, and chest discomfort.

4. Peptic Ulcer.

A peptic ulcer is any ulcer that occurs in the lining of the stomach, duodenum, or esophagus due to stomach acid. Peptic ulcers are further characterized as gastric, duodenal, and esophageal ulcers. All of these ulcers have comparable causes, including H. pylori infection, NSAID use, and lifestyle choices such as stress, smoking, and alcohol intake. Peptic ulcers are characterized by burning stomach pain, indigestion, and, in some cases, bleeding.

5. Stress Ulcer.

A stress ulcer is a peptic ulcer that develops due to extreme physiological stress. Stress ulcers, as opposed to other ulcers caused by bacterial infections or long-term pharmaceutical use, frequently form in people who are severely ill or have experienced serious physical damage, such as severe burns, brain injuries, or major surgery. These ulcers are more common in ICU patients and are hypothesized to be caused by diminished blood supply to the stomach and duodenum during periods of acute stress. If not addressed, stress ulcers can result in substantial gastrointestinal bleeding.

6. Refractory Ulcer.

A refractory ulcer does not heal or recur despite treatment. Peptic ulcers usually heal within a few months with the right drugs, such as proton pump inhibitors (PPIs) or H. pylori treatments. However, refractory ulcers persist despite treatment. Refractory ulcers can be caused by prolonged NSAID usage, poor H. pylori eradication, smoking, or underlying medical problems, including Zollinger-Ellison syndrome, which causes excessive stomach acid production.

NOTE

These stomach ulcers differ in location and etiology but are always caused by damage to the protective lining of the stomach, duodenum, or esophagus. Proper diagnosis and therapy are critical for controlling and healing ulcers efficiently.

Anatomy of the Digestive Tract

The digestive tract, commonly called the gastrointestinal (GI) tract, is a complicated system that processes food, absorbs nutrients, and removes waste. It starts at the mouth and finishes at the anus, and it is made up of numerous essential organs that work together to digest food, absorb nutrients, and eliminate waste. Understanding the anatomy of the digestive tract is critical, especially when looking at disorders like stomach ulcers, which arise in specific regions of the system.

Here's an overview of the main structures in the digestive tract:

1. MOUTH

The digestive process starts in the mouth when food is digested and broken down into smaller pieces via mastication (chewing). Salivary glands create enzymes like amylase, which begin to break down carbs. The tongue aids in food movement (now known as a bolus) to the back of the mouth for swallowing.

2. Esophagus.

The esophagus is a muscular tube that links the mouth and stomach. After swallowing, the bolus moves down the esophagus in a wave-like action known as peristalsis. The lower esophageal sphincter (LES) is a muscle valve at the lower end of the esophagus that limits food passage into the stomach and prevents stomach acid from flowing back up into the esophagus, which can lead to disorders such as esophageal ulcers.

3. Stomach

The stomach is a muscular, J-shaped organ essential for food digestion. It comprises digestive acids, primarily hydrochloric acid (HCl), and protein-digesting enzymes such as pepsin. The stomach generates mucus to protect its lining from the damaging effects of these high acids.

Food enters the stomach via the cardia and is churned into a semi-liquid called chyme. This procedure occurs in the body, the more extensive stomach section. The antrum, positioned near the stomach's lower end, propels chyme into the small intestine. The pyloric sphincter regulates the flow of chyme from the stomach to the small intestine.

If the stomach's mucus lining is damaged, acid can erode the stomach tissue and cause gastric ulcers.

4. Small intestine.

The small intestine is a long, coiled tube where most digesting and food absorption occurs. It is organized into three sections:

The duodenum is the first segment of the small intestine, where stomach chyme interacts with pancreatic digestive fluids and liver bile to complete food breakdown. Duodenal ulcers are common in this location because it is frequently exposed to acidic chyme.

The jejunum is the middle section of the small intestine that absorbs nutrients like carbs, proteins, and lipids.

The ileum is the final section of the small intestine, where vitamins (such as B12) and bile salts are absorbed before waste is transported to the large intestine.

5. Large intestine (colon)

The large intestine, or colon, absorbs water and electrolytes from the remaining indigestible food items and produces solid waste (stool). It contains the following:

Cecum: A pouch-like structure at the beginning of the big intestine.

Ascending, transverse, and descending colon: These regions absorb additional water and salt.

The sigmoid colon is the S-shaped last portion that connects to the rectum.

The large intestine is responsible for keeping the body hydrated and handling waste.

6. Rectum and Anus.

The rectum is the last portion of the large intestine and stores stool until it is ready to be evacuated. The anus is the hole via which stools exit the body. Muscles and sphincters regulate the discharge of waste during defecation.

Supporting organs

Several organs support the digestive process, even if they are not physically part of the gastrointestinal tract:

- The liver produces bile and aids in the digestion of lipids in the small intestine. It also detoxifies and preserves nutrients.
- The gallbladder stores the bile produced by the liver and discharges it into the small intestine as needed.

- Pancreas: The pancreas secretes enzymes that help digest proteins, lipids, and carbs. It also secretes insulin, which helps to control blood sugar levels.

How the Digestive Tract Relates to Stomach Ulcers

Understanding the anatomy of the digestive tract is critical when treating disorders such as stomach ulcers. Ulcers can appear in many locations of the digestive tract:

Gastric ulcers occur on the stomach lining.

Duodenal ulcers develop in the duodenum.

Acid reflux is a common cause of esophageal ulcers.

When the balance between stomach acid and the protective mucus lining is interrupted, ulcers can form, causing pain, bleeding, and other digestive issues.

Causes of Stomach Ulcers

1. Helicobacter pylori infection

H. pylori is a bacteria that can infect the stomach lining. It destroys the protective mucus layer, allowing stomach acid to irritate the lining and cause ulcer formation. This infection is common globally and is one of the leading causes of gastric and duodenal ulcers.

2. Nonsteroidal anti-inflammatory drugs (NSAIDs).

Long-term usage of NSAIDs like ibuprofen, aspirin, and naproxen can raise the chance of getting stomach ulcers. These drugs reduce the production of protective mucus in the stomach and may irritate the lining, making it more vulnerable to acid damage.

3. Increased Stomach Acid Production

Certain disorders, such as Zollinger-Ellison syndrome, cause excessive stomach acid production. This overproduction can overwhelm the stomach's defensive capabilities, leading to ulcers. Furthermore, stress and certain dietary variables may cause increased acid release.

4. Smoking.

Smoking is linked to an increased incidence of stomach ulcers. It decreases the formation of bicarbonate, which helps neutralize stomach acid and can also slow the healing of existing ulcers. Furthermore, smoking can raise stomach acid levels and worsen the consequences of H. pylori infections.

5. Alcohol consumption.

Excessive alcohol use can harm the stomach lining and raise acid levels. It can also cause inflammation of the stomach lining (gastritis), leading to ulcer formation. Individuals who consume large amounts of alcohol are more likely to develop gastric and duodenal ulcers.

6. Stress.

Stress is not a direct cause of stomach ulcers, although it can exacerbate pre-existing disorders. Stress can increase stomach acid production and lead to behaviors like poor eating habits or smoking, which raise the risk of ulcers. Chronic stress may also slow the healing of existing ulcers.

7. Spicy foods.

Spicy foods do not cause stomach ulcers but might irritate the stomach lining and worsen ulcer symptoms in certain people. Consuming spicy meals may cause further agony and misery in people who already have ulcers.

8. Family history of ulcers.

A family history of stomach ulcers can raise an individual's risk because genetic factors influence how the body makes stomach acid, responds to H. pylori infection, and maintains the stomach's protective lining. Genetic predispositions can affect the likelihood of acquiring ulcers.

9. Zollinger–Ellison Syndrome

Tumors in the pancreas or duodenum induce excessive release of the hormone gastrin, increasing stomach acid output. Excess acid can damage the stomach lining and cause ulcers.

10. Some medications (such as corticosteroids)

Corticosteroids, for example, can raise the risk of developing stomach ulcers when used over an extended period or at high doses. They can limit the stomach's ability to create mucus and slow the repair of existing ulcers, making the stomach lining more susceptible to acid damage.

Symptoms and Signs

Common symptoms include.

1. Burning stomach pain

A gnawing or burning sensation in the stomach, usually between meals or at night.

2. Bloating

A sensation of fullness or swelling in the abdomen, usually accompanied by discomfort.

3. Indigestion

General digestive discomfort, such as heartburn, gas, or nausea.

4. Nausea and vomiting.

Feeling sick to your stomach, which may lead to vomiting.

5. Loss of appetite

A decrease in the desire to eat is usually caused by pain or discomfort from eating.

6. Weight Loss

Unintentional weight loss is caused by reduced food intake due to ulcer pain.

Severe symptoms

1. Bleeding

This can have two forms:

- **Vomiting Blood:** The blood may be scarlet or look like coffee grounds.
- Black or tarry stools indicate bleeding in the upper gastrointestinal tract.

2. Severe abdominal pain.

Sudden, acute, or severe abdominal discomfort may indicate a perforated ulcer.

3. Fatigue

Feeling excessively tired or weak might be caused by blood loss or vitamin deficiencies.

4. Pale skin.

Chronic blood loss may cause anemia.

5. Shortness of breath.

Difficulty breathing, which can occur in extreme situations or after bleeding, causes significant blood loss.

6. Unexplained fever

If an infection or complication occurs, a fever may be present in addition to other symptoms.

When To Seek Medical Attention:

If you have any severe symptoms, such as vomiting blood, black stools, or severe abdominal discomfort, seek medical assistance right once. These could suggest complications like bleeding or perforation, which require immediate treatment.

Recognizing these symptoms and indicators early can lead to earlier diagnosis and treatment, considerably improving outcomes and preventing complications from stomach ulcers.

Diagnosis of Stomach Ulcers

1. Medical History and Physical Examination.

Medical History: The doctor will inquire about your symptoms, length, and intensity of pain, as well as any prior gastrointestinal difficulties, drug use (particularly NSAIDs), smoking, and alcohol consumption.

A physical examination may include palpating the abdomen for discomfort, bloating, or other abnormalities.

2. Endoscopy.

Upper Gastrointestinal (GI) endoscopy is a frequent and effective way to diagnose stomach ulcers. A thin, flexible tube with a camera (endoscope) is introduced through the mouth into the stomach. The doctor can immediately visualize the stomach lining and, if necessary, collect biopsies (tissue samples).

3. Imaging tests.

X-ray with Barium Swallow: During this test, the patient drinks a barium solution that coats the lining of the esophagus, stomach, and duodenum. X-ray scans are then obtained to detect any abnormalities, such as ulcers. This procedure is less frequently utilized than endoscopy.

A computed tomography (CT) scan of the abdomen can help visualize the digestive tract and detect issues such as perforation or obstruction.

4. Laboratory tests.

Blood tests may be performed to screen for anemia, which can indicate ulcer-related bleeding. Tests can also check for symptoms of illness or evaluate overall health.

Helicobacter Pylori Testing: There are several ways to test for H. pylori, including:

Breath Test: The patient drinks a urea-containing solution. If H. pylori is present, it will degrade the urea, producing carbon dioxide that can be detected in the breath.

Blood Test: This screens for antibodies to H. pylori but may not distinguish between previous and current infections.

Stool Test: A stool sample is examined for H. pylori antigens.

5. Biopsy

If an endoscopy discovers an ulcer, a biopsy may be performed to detect malignancy or H. pylori.

6. Additional tests.

In some circumstances, additional tests may be required to rule out problems or monitor stomach and intestine health.

Risk Factors and Who Is at Risk

Risk Factors for Stomach Ulcers:

1. Helicobacter pylori infection.

The presence of H. pylori bacteria is the leading cause of stomach ulcers. People with this illness are more likely to get ulcers.

2. The use of nonsteroidal anti-inflammatory drugs (NSAIDs)

Regular use of NSAIDs, such as ibuprofen, aspirin, and naproxen, can damage the stomach lining and raise the risk of ulcer formation.

3. Smoking

Tobacco use not only raises stomach acid levels but also affects the stomach's ability to heal, rendering smokers more vulnerable to ulcers.

4. Alcohol consumption

Heavy drinking can irritate the stomach lining and raise acid levels, increasing the risk of ulcers.

5. Stress

While stress does not cause ulcers, it can aggravate symptoms and lead to habits (such as improper eating) that raise ulcer risk.

6. Dietary Habits

A diet low in fruits and vegetables and high in processed foods may contribute to ulcer formation.

7. Family history of ulcers.

A genetic predisposition to stomach ulcers can raise the likelihood of acquiring them, mainly if the problem runs in the family.

8. Chronic illness.

Certain medical disorders, such as liver illness, renal disease, or chronic obstructive pulmonary disease (COPD), can increase the chance of developing ulcers.

9. Age

Older persons are more likely to develop ulcers, which is attributed in part to decreased mucus production and increasing usage of drugs such as NSAIDs.

10. Prior history of ulcers.

Individuals who have previously experienced ulcers are more prone to acquire them again.

Who is at risk?

- Individuals with H. pylori Infection: Anyone infected with this bacteria, especially in areas with excellent prevalence rates.
- Long-term NSAID users are those who use them regularly to treat illnesses like arthritis or chronic pain.
- **Smokers**: People who smoke or are exposed to secondhand smoke.
- Heavy alcohol consumers are those who consume significant amounts of alcohol regularly.

- **Individuals Under Significant Stress:** Those stressed out due to personal, professional, or health concerns.

- Older adults, specifically those aged 60 and up.

- **People with a Family History of Ulcers:** Those genetically predisposed to stomach ulcers.

- **Patients with Chronic Diseases:** People with chronic illnesses may be at a higher risk because of drugs or the stress of managing their symptoms.

CHAPTER TWO: Diet and Nutrition for Ulcer Healing

In this chapter, we'll look at how the foods you eat can aggravate and heal stomach ulcers. Diet is more than simply food; it may help your body heal or cause more agony. Throughout this chapter, you'll discover how to make food choices that encourage ulcer recovery and overall digestive health.

We'll start by discussing foods to avoid, such as hot, acidic, and fatty foods, before moving on to healing foods high in fiber, probiotics, and omega-3 fatty acids. These foods will help calm the stomach lining and minimize inflammation. You'll also learn about the benefits of eating small, frequent meals, which can help prevent acid production and gastrointestinal irritation.

Next, we'll look at the nutritional components that aid recovery, such as dietary fiber, antioxidants, probiotics, and water. Each ingredient helps to mend and strengthen your digestive tract, laying the groundwork for long-term ulcer treatment.

We'll also discuss vitamins and natural therapies, such as aloe vera, licorice root, and herbal teas, which have been proven to have additional therapeutic properties. These solutions might supplement your diet by naturally soothing and healing ulcers.

As we progress, you'll receive advice on creating a balanced diet plan that meets your needs, such as a meal plan, portion management recommendations, and healthy snacking options. You'll also learn to analyze your dietary tolerances by maintaining a meal diary and noting foods that cause discomfort or acid reflux.

Finally, we'll talk about transitioning to a long-term gut-healthy diet by including healing foods into your daily routine and reaping the long-term advantages of a well-balanced diet that promotes digestive health.

This chapter will provide you with the knowledge and resources you need to make informed, effective decisions that will help you manage your ulcer, reduce symptoms, and adopt a healthy lifestyle.

The Role of Diet in Managing Ulcers

Diet is an essential factor in controlling and healing stomach ulcers. Ulcers arise when the lining of the stomach or duodenum (the first part of the small intestine) is destroyed, most usually caused by the bacterium Helicobacter pylori or long-term use of nonsteroidal anti-inflammatory medicines. While drugs like proton pump inhibitors (PPIs) and antibiotics may be used to treat ulcers, dietary adjustments might help to promote healing and keep symptoms from worsening. Proper diet choices can help preserve the stomach lining, reduce irritation, and speed up recovery, but certain foods might worsen the ulcer and create further agony.

Foods to Avoid: Spicy, Acidic, and Fatty

Learning which foods to avoid is one of the first stages in diet-based ulcer management. Certain meals can release stomach acid, irritate the stomach lining, or slow the healing of an ulcer. Avoiding these foods is critical for lowering inflammation and keeping ulcer symptoms from worsening.

1. Spicy foods.

Spicy foods are frequently blamed for ulcers, even though they do not directly cause ulcer formation. However, they can worsen pre-existing ulcers by irritating the stomach lining and boosting acid production. Spicy peppers, chili powder, curry, and spicy sauces may aggravate the burning sensation caused by ulcers.

Patients with ulcers should limit or eliminate spicy meals to avoid exacerbating symptoms.

2. Acidic foods.

Acidic meals such as citrus fruits (oranges, lemons, grapefruits), tomatoes, and vinegar can raise stomach acid and exacerbate ulcers. These foods may cause acid reflux or worsen the burning sensation accompanying ulcers. While tiny amounts of acidic foods may not impact everyone similarly, those with ulcers should monitor their tolerance levels and avoid eating considerable amounts.

3. Fatty foods.

High-fat foods inhibit digestion and can increase acid production in the stomach, potentially aggravating an ulcer. Fatty foods like fried chicken, heavy creams, greasy fast food, and full-fat dairy products should be avoided. Not only do they boost acid production, but they also cause bloating and discomfort, making it more difficult for the stomach to consume food efficiently. Instead, lean proteins and low-fat dairy can be more stomach-friendly options.

Other foods and beverages to avoid are:

- *Caffeine:* Found in coffee, tea, and chocolate, caffeine can increase stomach acid production and cause symptoms such as heartburn or indigestion.
- Alcohol irritates the stomach lining and slows ulcer healing. Therefore, it's important to restrict or eliminate alcohol consumption.
- Carbonated drinks like soda and sparkling water can induce bloating and raise stomach pressure, resulting in acid reflux and pain.

Healing Foods (Fiber, Probiotics, and Omega-3)

While some foods should be avoided, others can calm the stomach lining and help ulcers recover. These foods are high in fiber, probiotics, and omega-3 fatty acids, which help to promote digestive health, reduce inflammation, and restore the balance of healthy bacteria in the gut.

1. Fiber-rich foods.

Dietary fiber promotes gut health and helps to prevent ulcers. Fiber reduces the amount of acid in the stomach and may aid in the repair of its lining. High-fiber diets, particularly those high in soluble fiber, can help avoid bloating and indigestion by facilitating easier digestion.

Examples of fiber-rich diets useful for ulcers are:

- Oatmeal, brown rice, and whole wheat bread contain soluble fiber, which absorbs excess stomach acid and relieves inflammation.
- Legumes are high in fiber and protein.
- **Fruits and vegetables:** Apples, pears, carrots, sweet potatoes, and bananas are soothing on the stomach and provide essential nutrients without causing excessive acid production.

2. Probiotics and Fermented foods.

Probiotics are living bacteria that help maintain a healthy gut flora. They aid in treating H. pylori infections, one of the primary causes of ulcers, and can also improve the body's healing ability. Consuming probiotic-rich meals helps restore the natural balance of bacteria in the stomach and small intestine, which can aid patients suffering from ulcers.

Probiotic-rich foods include:

- Yogurt (with living cultures), particularly those with Lactobacillus and Bifidobacterium strains.
- **Kefir:** A fermented dairy drink rich in probiotics that assist digestion.
- Sauerkraut and kimchi are fermented vegetables that contain helpful microorganisms for digestive health.

3. Omega 3 Fatty Acids

Omega-3 fatty acids have anti-inflammatory properties and can help to relieve stomach lining inflammation. They also promote healing by lowering inflammation throughout the digestive tract. Omega-3s are present in:

- **Fatty Fish:** Salmon, mackerel, and sardines are high in omega-3.
- **Flaxseeds and Chia Seeds:** These plant-based sources of omega-3 fatty acids are easily incorporated into smoothies, porridge, and yogurt.
- **Walnuts:** Another excellent plant-based source of omega-3 fats that you may incorporate into your regular diet.

The Value of Small, Frequent Meals

When treating stomach ulcers, how you eat is as important as what you consume. Eating small, frequent meals throughout the day can help lower stomach acid, avoid bloating, and relieve strain on the stomach lining. Large meals frequently increase stomach acid production, irritating the ulcer and impeding healing. Smaller, more manageable portions help to control acid levels and lessen the incidence of acid reflux.

Advantages of Eating Small, Frequent Meals:

- **Reduced stomach acid production:** Smaller meals require less digestive acid, benefiting the stomach lining.
- **Consistent Nutrient Intake:** Frequent meals eliminate extended gaps between meals, which can cause acid production when the stomach is empty. This provides a regular supply of nutrients throughout the day.
- **Less pressure on the stomach.** Large meals can strain the stomach, causing acid reflux and pain. Small meals lessen this pressure, lowering the likelihood of discomfort.

Timing of meals

It's also critical to time your meals correctly. Eating your final meal at least three hours before bedtime allows your stomach to process the food before lying down, lowering your chances of acid reflux and discomfort at night. Eating deliberately and adequately can also help with digestion and lessen the likelihood of post-meal pain.

Nutritional Components for Ulcer Recovery

Nutrition is essential in rehabilitating stomach ulcers. Certain nutrients can help mend the stomach lining, reduce inflammation, and improve overall gut health. The appropriate dietary components not only help with healing but also prevent ulcers from recurring. Let's look at these crucial dietary components for ulcer recovery.

Dietary Fiber: Its Role in Gut Health

Dietary fiber is crucial for digestive health and helps manage ulcers. There are two types of fiber: soluble fiber and insoluble fiber. Both contribute to better gut health, but soluble fiber is perfect for stomach ulcer patients.

Advantages of Fiber for Ulcer Recovery:

- *Reduces Stomach Acid Levels:* Soluble fiber, found in foods such as oats, lentils, and fruits, helps absorb excess stomach acid, preventing ulcer aggravation and promoting healing. Soluble fiber slows digestion, which minimizes acid production and causes less stomach lining discomfort.

- *Promotes Healthy Digestion:* Fiber promotes smooth digestion by keeping the gut regular and reducing constipation. This is essential for avoiding pressure buildup in the stomach, which can aggravate ulcer symptoms.

- *Improves gut health:* A high-fiber diet nourishes the gut's beneficial bacteria, promoting a healthy microbiome and improving overall digestive health. A healthy gut flora can help to avoid future infections and repair ulcers faster.

Sources of dietary fiber:

- *Oatmeal:* A soluble fiber-rich diet that soothes ulcer patients.
- Fruits and vegetables: Apples, carrots, sweet potatoes, bananas, and pears are easy on the stomach and include fiber and necessary nutrients.
- *Whole Grains:* Fiber-rich foods like brown rice, quinoa, and whole wheat bread can help keep your gut healthy.
- *Legumes:* Lentils, chickpeas, and beans are high in fiber and protein, making them ideal for ulcer rehabilitation.

Antioxidants and Their Benefits (Vitamin A, C, E)

Antioxidants protect the body from free radicals. They help to repair and preserve the stomach lining and reduce inflammation caused by ulcers. The essential antioxidant vitamins, Vitamin A, Vitamin C, and Vitamin E, are very effective for ulcer healing.

1. Vitamin A has a role in healing by maintaining the stomach's mucosal lining, which serves as a barrier against acid. It also promotes tissue regeneration, accelerating the healing process.

Sources include carrots, sweet potatoes, spinach, kale, and liver.

2. Vitamin C plays a crucial role in healing by stimulating the immune system and combating H. pylori infections, a leading cause of ulcers. It also helps to produce collagen, a protein that aids in the repair of damaged tissues in the stomach lining.

Citrus fruits (e.g., oranges and grapefruits), strawberries, bell peppers, broccoli, and Brussels sprouts.

3. Vitamin E's Healing Role: Vitamin E's anti-inflammatory effects protect the stomach lining from acid damage and oxidative stress. It can minimize inflammation and promote speedier healing.

Sources include nuts, seeds, avocados, and leafy green vegetables.

Integrating these antioxidant-rich foods into your diet can encourage faster healing of the stomach lining and prevent further oxidative damage.

Probiotics and Fermented Food

Probiotics are living bacteria and yeasts that promote intestinal health. These microorganisms help balance the gut microbiome, lowering the number of dangerous bacteria such as Helicobacter pylori, which is frequently the underlying cause of stomach ulcers. Probiotic-rich meals can aid in ulcer healing by aiding digestion and bolstering the body's natural defenses against infection.

Benefits of Probiotics:

- *Combat H. pylori Infection:* Probiotics help reduce H. pylori colonization in the stomach, accelerating ulcer healing and preventing recurrence.
- *Support Digestive Health:* Probiotics establish a healthy balance of good bacteria in the digestive tract, reducing inflammation and speeding up the healing of the stomach lining.
- Probiotics stimulate the immune system, allowing it to combat harmful germs more efficiently.

Sources of probiotics:

- Yogurt (containing living cultures) is an excellent source of probiotics such as Lactobacillus and Bifidobacterium, which enhance digestive health.
- Kefir is a fermented dairy product rich in probiotics that promote gut health.
- Sauerkraut and kimchi are fermented vegetables rich in beneficial bacteria that assist digestion and reduce inflammation.

- Miso and tempeh are fermented soy products that contain beneficial bacteria and improve ulcer healing.
- Incorporating probiotic-rich foods into your diet can help to mend the stomach lining and restore balance to your digestive system.

Hydration and the Function of Fluids

Staying hydrated is essential for overall health and is especially helpful in ulcer management. Adequate fluid intake helps to maintain the stomach's protective mucus lining, keeping it intact and preventing excess acid from causing additional harm. Water is the best fluid for hydration, but other beverages that promote ulcer healing can also be included in the diet.

Hydration benefits include maintaining a healthy mucus layer, which protects the stomach lining from acid damage.

Proper fluid consumption aids digestion by breaking down food and facilitating easy digestion, decreasing bloating and discomfort.

Drinking water helps eliminate toxins from the body, which improves general digestive health and ulcer repair.

Fluids to Prioritize:

- *Water:* Drinking enough water throughout the day helps to keep you hydrated and supports the stomach's protective mucus layer.
- *Herbal Teas:* Chamomile, ginger, and licorice root teas are known to relax the digestive system and reduce inflammation, making them excellent choices for ulcer patients.
- Aloe vera juice has anti-inflammatory effects and helps soothe the stomach lining, allowing ulcers to heal faster.

- *Coconut water:* This natural beverage is high in electrolytes and gentle on the stomach, making it an excellent choice for staying hydrated without irritating the ulcer.

Fluids to Avoid:

- Avoid caffeinated drinks such as coffee, black tea, and sodas, which might raise stomach acid and exacerbate ulcers.
- *Alcohol:* Alcohol can harm the stomach lining and should be avoided, particularly during ulcer rehabilitation.

Staying hydrated with the correct fluids can help digestion, protect the stomach lining, and speed up the healing of ulcers.

Supplements and Natural Remedies

Natural medicines and vitamins can help stomach ulcers heal when used with a well-balanced diet. These therapies reduce inflammation, promote tissue repair, and soothe the stomach lining.

Aloe Vera and Licorice Root for Ulcer Healing.

- *Aloe vera:* Aloe vera is known for its anti-inflammatory and relaxing characteristics, which can help relieve stomach lining irritation. It improves healing and can help to reduce stomach acid, making it useful for ulcer repair.
- *Licorice Root:* Deglycyrrhizinated licorice (DGL) is a type of licorice treated to eliminate components that can elevate blood pressure. DGL has been demonstrated to protect the stomach lining by boosting mucus production, which shields the stomach from acid and allows ulcers to heal more quickly.

Advantages of Zinc and L-Glutamine

- *Zinc:* This mineral is necessary for wound healing and tissue restoration. Zinc supplementation can increase stomach lining regeneration, resulting in speedier ulcer healing.

- L-glutamine is an amino acid essential for gut health. It helps mend the stomach lining and can protect against future acid damage. It is especially helpful in aiding the repair of the intestinal wall and decreasing inflammation.

Herbal Teas: Chamomile, Green Tea, Ginger

- Chamomile tea is believed to relax the digestive system. It reduces inflammation, soothes the stomach lining, and may even alleviate acid reflux symptoms, relieving individuals with ulcers.
- Green tea is high in antioxidants, notably catechins, which can lower inflammation and help fight Helicobacter pylori, a common cause of ulcers. Its anti-inflammatory characteristics also help to mend the stomach lining.
- **Ginger Tea:** Ginger is recognized for its digestive properties. It reduces nausea, improves digestion, and contains anti-inflammatory qualities that may aid in ulcer healing by relieving stomach irritation.

Creating a Balanced Diet Plan

A balanced meal plan is essential in controlling stomach ulcers and aiding healing. The idea is to eat meals that calm the stomach lining, reduce acid production, and promote healing while providing appropriate nutrients. A balanced diet for ulcer patients should focus on mild, readily digestible meals while avoiding those that irritate the stomach. This includes adding fiber-rich foods, lean proteins, healthy fats, and natural anti-inflammatory components. Pay attention to portion quantities, meal timing, and healthy snacking habits to avoid overburdening the digestive system.

Sample 7-Day Meal Plan for Ulcer Patients.

A well-planned meal plan ensures you obtain enough nutrients to encourage healing while avoiding common ulcer triggers such as spicy, acidic, or fatty meals. Here is a sample 7-day diet plan designed exclusively for ulcer patients.

Day 1:

Breakfast: Oatmeal with honey and sliced banana.

Lunch: grilled chicken salad with lush greens, cucumbers, and an olive oil dressing.

Dinner: Baked Salmon with Steamed Carrots and Brown Rice

Snack: Apple slices and a tiny handful of almonds.

Day 2:

Breakfast: Scrambled eggs with spinach and whole wheat bread.

Lunch: lentil soup and soft bread.

Dinner: grilled turkey breast, quinoa, and sautéed zucchini.

Snack: Greek yogurt with honey.

Day 3:

Breakfast: Smoothie with almond milk, blueberries, and flaxseeds.

Lunch: Tuna salad with avocado in a whole wheat wrap.

Dinner: Broiled cod with mashed sweet potatoes and steamed broccoli.

Snack: unsweetened applesauce.

Day 4:

Breakfast: Cottage cheese with sliced pears.

Lunch: Brown rice, black beans, and steamed spinach

Dinner: Grilled chicken, quinoa, and vegetable stir-fry

Snack: Carrot sticks and hummus

Day 5

Breakfast: Whole grain cereal with almond milk and strawberries.

Lunch: turkey and avocado sandwich on whole wheat toast.

Dinner: baked tofu, steamed green beans, and wild rice

Snack: One banana with a tiny handful of sunflower seeds.

Day 6:

Breakfast: Smoothie with Greek yogurt, mango, and chia seeds.

Lunch: Grilled shrimp with couscous and sautéed greens.

Dinner: Roasted chicken with sweet potatoes and steamed asparagus.

Snack: handful of unsalted walnuts.

Day 7:

Breakfast: Consisted of soft-boiled eggs, whole-grain bread, and a tiny melon.

Lunch: Quinoa salad with cherry tomatoes, cucumbers, and feta cheese.

Dinner: Baked trout, roasted Brussels sprouts, and brown rice

Snack: Low-fat cheese and whole-grain crackers.

This sample meal plan contains a variety of lean proteins, fiber-rich grains, veggies, and soothing snacks that can help with stomach ulcers. The meals are intended to be soft on the stomach, with minimum usage of acid-producing or irritating components.

Portion Control and Meal Timing.

Portion control and meal timing are critical elements in ulcer care. Large meals can cause increased stomach acid production, worsening ulcer symptoms. As a result, eating smaller, more frequent meals throughout the day is essential for avoiding discomfort and aiding the digestive process.

- **Portion Control Tips:** Eat smaller meals more frequently. Instead of eating three large meals, aim for 5-6 smaller meals spread out throughout the day. This stops the stomach from creating too much acid at once.

- **Avoid overeating:** Eating until you're total puts additional strain on the stomach, forcing it to create more acid and possibly resulting in reflux or pain.

- **Use Smaller Plates:** Smaller dishes allow you to reduce your portion sizes without feeling deprived naturally. Fill your plate with meals high in nutrients and good for your ulcers.

- **Chew food thoroughly:** Chewing thoroughly aids in the breakdown of food and facilitates digestion, lowering the risk of bloating and indigestion.

Meal Timing Tips

- **Avoid skipping meals:** Skipping meals causes the stomach to create too much acid, exacerbating ulcers. Eat at regular intervals to keep stomach acid production consistent.

- **Avoid Late-Night Eating:** Eating just before bedtime might cause acid reflux and discomfort. Try to eat your last meal at least 2-3 hours before lying down.

- **Keep Snacks on Hand:** Eating healthy snacks in between meals will keep your stomach from becoming overly empty, which can cause symptoms. Concentrate on ulcer-friendly foods such as yogurt, bananas, and whole grains.

Snacking Tips: Healthy Alternatives

Snacking can be essential to an ulcer-friendly diet, mainly if you eat smaller, more frequent meals. However, the snacks you eat might significantly impact how well you manage your symptoms. It is critical to choose foods that relax the stomach and avoid those that may cause acid production or irritation.

Healthy Snacking Tip:

- Choose Fiber-Rich Snacks to regulate digestion and lower stomach acid levels. Snacks like whole grain crackers, bananas, and oatmeal might assist in regulating your digestive system.

- **Incorporate Probiotic-Rich Foods:** Probiotics support gut health and can reduce ulcer-related inflammation. Consider munching on live-cultured yogurt or kefir.

- **Avoid acidic snacks:** Citrus fruits, tomato-based snacks, and spicy dips should be avoided because they irritate the stomach lining and exacerbate ulcer symptoms.

- **Include Lean Proteins:** Hard-boiled eggs, a small portion of turkey, or a handful of nuts (such as almonds or walnuts) will provide long-lasting energy without overburdening your digestive system.

Snack Ideas For Ulcer Patients:

- **Low-Fat Yogurt with Honey:** This yogurt contains probiotics to enhance digestive health and add sweetness without upsetting the stomach.

- Bananas are gentle on the stomach and high in fiber and potassium, which can help regulate acid production.

- Whole-grain crackers with Hummus: Hummus is high in fiber and protein, while the crackers contain slow-digesting carbohydrates.

- **Apples with Peanut Butter:** Apples are high-fiber fruits, and combining them with peanut butter adds protein and healthy fats to balance the snack.

- **Carrot Sticks with Cottage Cheese:** Carrots are high in fiber and vitamins, while cottage cheese contains protein and is easy to digest.

- **Oatmeal with Berries:** Oatmeal soothes the stomach, and adding berries adds antioxidants and fiber, making it a nutritious snack.

Assessing Personal Food Tolerances

Assessing personal food tolerances is critical for managing stomach ulcers because everyone reacts differently to meals. Understanding how your body responds to different foods allows you to adapt your diet to prevent triggers and encourage healing.

Keep a Food Diary

Keeping a food diary is one of the most effective methods for determining which foods cause pain. By documenting your eating habits and noting any symptoms that arise, you can notice patterns over time. Keep track of every meal, snack, and drink you consume, as well as the time and accompanying symptoms such as pain, bloating, or reflux. This will help you identify foods that may be causing your ulcer symptoms.

Addressing Reflux and Acid Production

Reflux and excessive acid production can exacerbate ulcer symptoms; therefore, controlling them is critical. Small, regular meals might help keep the stomach from growing overly full and causing acid reflux. Avoid lying down immediately after eating, and choose low-acid, non-spicy foods. Drinking plenty of water and avoiding caffeinated or carbonated beverages can help keep acid production under control.

Identifying Trigger Foods

Through tracking and observation, you'll begin to distinguish trigger foods—those that aggravate symptoms. Spices, citrus fruits, coffee, alcohol, and fatty or fried foods are all common triggers. Once recognized, cutting or limiting your intake can significantly relieve ulcer symptoms and improve digestive comfort.

Transitioning to a Long-Term Gut-Healthy Diet

Once your stomach ulcer has begun to heal, it is critical to adopt a long-term gut-healthy diet to maintain digestive health, avoid new ulcers, and promote overall well-being. This transition should be centered on incorporating healing foods into your daily routine, reducing past trigger foods, and comprehending the long-term benefits of a gut-friendly diet. Making these lifestyle changes permanent can improve your digestive health and lessen the likelihood of ulcers returning.

Adding Healing Foods to Your Routine

Healing foods should become a regular part of your daily diet to help maintain gut health and healing. These meals lower inflammation, support good digestion, and protect the stomach lining from injury.

Steps for Integrating Healing Foods:

- *Start with fiber-rich foods:* Incorporate fiber into each meal. Soluble fiber found in oats, fruits, vegetables, and legumes can assist in absorbing excess acid and calm the stomach lining. Fiber also promotes regular bowel motions and feeds beneficial microorganisms in the stomach.

- *Probiotics:* Continue to consume probiotic-rich foods like yogurt, kefir, sauerkraut, and other fermented foods to maintain a healthy balance of gut bacteria. Probiotics promote digestion and help protect the stomach lining from dangerous bacteria such as H. pylori.

- *Include omega-3 fatty acids:* Salmon, flaxseeds, chia seeds, and walnuts contain omega-3 fatty acids with anti-inflammatory qualities. Regularly consuming these foods can help lower intestinal inflammation and improve healing.

- *Hydrate with Healing Beverages:* Herbal teas (including chamomile, ginger, and licorice root) and water should be part of your regular hydration regimen.

These liquids are mild on the stomach and can relieve discomfort while aiding digestion.

- *Focus on Lean Proteins:* Chicken, turkey, fish, tofu, and lentils are more digestible and do not cause acid formation like fatty meats. Incorporating these into meals will give essential nutrients without irritating the stomach.

Meal Planning for Success:

- ***Gradually incorporate new foods:*** Introduce these therapeutic meals gradually into your daily routine to allow your digestive system to adjust. Begin with tiny servings, gradually increasing them over time.

- *Rotate Foods to Avoid Boredom:* Alternate your fiber, protein, and probiotic sources to keep meals exciting and avoid reverting to less healthy habits. Experiment with different fruits, vegetables, grains, and protein sources to ensure variety and balanced nutrition.

Moderation of Past Triggers

While you may have removed some trigger foods during your ulcer's healing period, shifting to a long-term diet does not require you to avoid all of them indefinitely. Moderation and careful reintroduction can allow you to eat some of your old favorites without risking your digestive health.

Steps for Moderation:

- *Gradually reintroduce trigger foods:* Begin with tiny portions of things you used to avoid, such as spicy, acidic, or fatty foods. Pay close attention to your body's reactions. If no symptoms develop, you may be able to consume these items in moderation.

- *Limit Portion Sizes:* If you discover that particular foods still cause slight discomfort, you do not have to avoid them altogether. Instead, keep the portions small and avoid eating these items too frequently. For example, instead of making spicy food a regular part of your diet, have it occasionally.

- *Time Your Meals Carefully:* Avoid eating potential trigger foods late at night or on an empty stomach, as these situations might increase acid production. Consume these meals as part of a balanced diet to decrease the impact on the stomach.

- *Choose Healthier Alternatives:* If you miss the flavor of trigger foods such as fried or spicy dishes, look into healthier options. For example, instead of deep-frying dishes, try baking or grilling them, and replace spicy ingredients with milder, gut-friendly herbs such as turmeric or ginger.

Foods to keep in check:

- *Caffeine and alcohol:* Both can increase acid production and irritate the stomach lining. Limit your intake of these substances, or opt for decaffeinated and non-alcoholic alternatives wherever possible.

- Spicy foods can trigger, so use milder seasonings and spices to lessen their impact.

- *Acidic Fruits:* While citrus fruits and tomatoes can still be enjoyed, they should be consumed in moderation or replaced with less acidic options such as bananas and melons.

Long-Term Advantages of A Gut-Friendly Diet

Transitioning to a long-term gut-healthy diet has various benefits in addition to ulcer management. Eating a diet high in healing foods and avoiding irritants may support your digestive health and well-being.

Benefits for Digestive Health:

- A gut-healthy diet promotes a balanced intestinal environment, reduces inflammation, and supports stomach lining regeneration, minimizing the risk of recurrent ulcers.

- *Better Digestive Function:* Eating enough fiber and probiotics encourages regular bowel movements, decreases bloating, and keeps your digestive tract running smoothly.

- *Improved Gut Microbiome:* A well-balanced diet high in probiotics and fiber promotes the growth of good bacteria, which aids digestion, boosts immune function, and lowers the risk of illnesses such as H. pylori.

Overall Health Benefits:

- *Anti-inflammatory Effects:* A gut-friendly diet contains omega-3 fatty acids, antioxidants, and other anti-inflammatory components that help reduce systemic inflammation, which benefits not only your gut but also your heart and brain.

- *Increased Energy and Nutrient Absorption:* Promoting healthy digestion allows your body to absorb nutrients more effectively, resulting in higher energy levels, increased immunological function, and overall wellness.

- *Weight Management:* A well-balanced, gut-healthy diet rich in whole foods, lean proteins, and fiber will help you maintain a healthy weight without resorting to restrictive diets.

Emotional and Mental Wellbeing:

- *Reduced Gut Stress:* A diet that reduces gut irritation also benefits mental health, as digestive discomfort can cause anxiety, stress, and a lower quality of life. A gut-friendly diet can help you manage symptoms and feel more at peace in your daily life.

- *Sustained Lifestyle Changes:* The benefits go far beyond ulcer treatment once your body adapts to a gut-healthy diet. A well-balanced diet can have long-term benefits for your physical and emotional health, making it more straightforward to stick with these practices.

This chapter covers essential lifestyle modifications that can significantly enhance the treatment of stomach ulcers and promote long-term healing. Dietary changes are only one aspect of ulcer therapy; other strategies include stress management, getting the recommended amount of exercise, and changing bad habits that could worsen your disease.

We'll begin by discussing the connection between stress and ulcers and offering coping mechanisms to promote healing, such as mindfulness, meditation, and relaxation techniques. Additionally, you'll learn how exercise, exceptionally mild exercises, can help with digestion without causing symptoms to worsen.

We'll also discuss habit management, with an emphasis on cutting back on bad habits like drinking alcohol, smoking, and consuming caffeine. The chapter will highlight the value of support networks and mental health and provide advice on how to get emotional support, get treatment, and create a community to make long-lasting lifestyle changes.

This chapter concludes by offering helpful advice on incorporating ulcer management into your everyday life, from developing routines and food plans to monitoring your health with routine examinations and modifying your treatment plan as necessary. These all-encompassing lifestyle changes will help you manage ulcers more effectively and enhance your general health.

Stress Management and Ulcer Healing

Since stress can majorly impact digestive health, managing stress is essential to ulcer repair. Stress can worsen symptoms and slow the healing process, even though it may not be the actual cause of ulcers. Stress can impair the body's capacity to heal the stomach lining, increase the production of stomach acid, and interfere with digestion. Therefore, it is crucial to help ulcer repair by implementing stress management practices into your everyday routine.

Stress's Effect on Digestive Health

Stress impacts the digestive system in several ways. Stress causes the body to release chemicals like cortisol and adrenaline, which can produce more stomach acid. This increased stomach acid can irritate the lining, making ulcer sufferers uncomfortable. Chronic stress can also result in unhealthy eating patterns, smoking, or binge drinking, all of which exacerbate ulcers.

Stress also impacts the gut-brain axis, which connects the brain and digestive system. Prolonged stress can worsen ulcer diseases by slowing digestion, causing bloating, and causing more acute symptoms like indigestion or acid reflux.

Techniques for Meditation and Mindfulness

Meditation and mindfulness are effective strategies for lowering stress and enhancing ulcer care. These techniques improve general well-being, lessen the body's stress reaction, and soothe the mind.

The advantages of meditation and mindfulness for the healing of ulcers

- *Reduces Production of Stomach Acid:* Mindfulness and meditation can help minimize excess stomach acid production by lowering stress hormone levels.

- *Enhances Digestive Function:* By promoting mindful eating, mindfulness practices help improve digestion and avoid overeating, a significant cause of ulcers.

- *Encourages Relaxation:* By assisting the body in transitioning from a "fight-or-flight" state to a more relaxed one, meditation improves the efficiency of the digestive system.

Methods to Try:

- *Mindful Breathing:* Do slow, deep breathing exercises to relax your body and mind. Pay attention to your breath as you inhale and exhale to relieve tension and stress.

- *Body Scan Meditation:* This method is mentally going over your entire body, from head to toe, finding any tense spots, and then relaxing intently to release those tensions.

- *Guided Meditation:* Use meditation applications or audio guides to help you relax deeply and concentrate on peaceful imagery. This will help you release tension.

Yoga and Calming Activities

Yoga is an excellent workout for ulcer repair and stress reduction. In contrast to intense exercise, yoga uses deep breathing, relaxation techniques, and gentle motions to promote digestive health without exacerbating ulcer symptoms. Yoga increases circulation and lowers stress hormones, both of which assist the stomach lining repair.

Yoga's advantages for healing ulcers

- *Reduces Stress and Anxiety:* Yoga helps reduce acid production and stress by promoting relaxation through gentle postures and controlled breathing.

- *Enhances Digestion:* Several yoga positions stimulate the digestive organs, helping improve digestion and lessen discomfort or bloating.

- *Promotes Relaxation:* After yoga practice, relaxation poses help calm the nervous system and relieve tense muscles, which can lessen pain associated with ulcers.

Try These Yoga Pose Ideas:

The child's pose (Balasana) is a soft, healing pose that promotes deep breathing and relaxation. It lowers stress and soothes the digestive tract.

The Cat-Cow Pose (Marjaryasana-Bitilasana) helps digestion by gently stimulating the organs and stretching the abdominal muscles.

The pose known as "seated forward bend" (Paschimottanasana) helps people relax and stretch their lower back and digestive organs, making them feel less bloated and uncomfortable.

Apart from yoga, basic relaxation techniques such as progressive muscle relaxation (PMR) can aid in the body's stress release. PMR helps lower stress and encourage general relaxation by methodically tensing and relaxing various muscle groups.

Physical Activity and Its Role in Gut Health

Physical activity is essential for managing stomach ulcers and preserving gut health. Frequent movement helps balance the body's processes, lowers stress, and enhances digestion. The appropriate forms of exercise can promote healing and lessen discomfort for those with ulcers. However, since strenuous workouts can exacerbate symptoms and prolong recovery, selecting exercises that do not place an undue amount of strain on the body is crucial.

Mild Exercises: Yoga, Swimming, and Walking

People with ulcers benefit significantly from gentle exercises. Due to their moderate impact, these activities improve digestion, lower stress levels, and make the stomach comfortable. Without undue strain on the digestive system, they promote digestion, increase circulation, and enhance general well-being.

1. Strolling/Walking

Walking is one of the most accessible yet most beneficial types of exercise for gut health. Walking for 20 to 30 minutes after meals promotes digestion, keeps food from remaining in the stomach for too long, and lessens bloating and discomfort. Additionally, walking increases blood flow to the digestive system, which supports improved stomach lining function and healing.

2. Swimming

Another low-impact activity that is good for the digestive system and easy on the stomach is swimming. Without creating the extreme strain that might worsen ulcer symptoms, swimming's rhythmic motions help lower stress, increase circulation, and improve general physical fitness. Additionally, swimming encourages relaxation, which aids in the body's recovery.

3. Yoga

Yoga is perfect for stress management and digestive health since it incorporates controlled breathing, moderate movement, and stretching. Yoga poses that gently massage the abdominal organs, such as Twists, Cat-Cow, and Child's Pose, improve digestion and lessen bloating. Yoga also helps reduce stress hormones, stopping the stomach lining from irritation and producing too much acid.

Steer clear of intense exercises that exacerbate symptoms.

Exercise is crucial, but not all types of exercise are suitable for people with ulcers. Running, lifting hefty weights, or doing vigorous aerobic activities are high-intensity workouts that might exacerbate ulcer symptoms and slow recovery. Exercises like these frequently raise the production of stress hormones, which increases stomach acid levels and irritates the lining.

Reasons Not to Engage in High-Intensity Exercise:

- *Elevated Production of Stomach Acid:* Excessive stomach acid production might aggravate pre-existing ulcers due to elevated cortisol and adrenaline levels from high-intensity exercise.

- *Digestive pain:* High-impact activities may cause the belly to shift jarringly, resulting in bloating, acid reflux, or other discomfort. Heavy lifting and vigorous abdominal exercises might also strain the digestive system.

- *Delays in Recovery:* When the body is overexerted, it may take longer to heal the stomach lining since it is more concerned with recovering from physical stress.

Instead, concentrate on mild, moderate activities that support general well-being without taxing the digestive system.

Movement Is Essential for Digestion

Maintaining a healthy digestive system requires regular exercise. Food moves more quickly when the digestive system moves, lowering the chance of bloating, gas, and constipation. Furthermore, exercise strengthens the gastrointestinal tract's muscles, which improves digestion and promotes gut health in general.

Movement's Benefits for Digestion

- *Better Bowel Movements:* Constipation, a typical problem for persons with digestive issues, can be avoided, and bowel movements can be regulated with exercise, exceptionally light, and regular activity like walking.

- *Improved Blood Flow to Digestive Organs:* Exercise improves circulation, guaranteeing that the intestines and stomach get enough oxygen and nutrients—essential for recovery and optimum performance.

- *Reduction of Bloating and Gas:* Regular movement makes food pass through the digestive tract more quickly and minimizes intestinal fermentation, lowering the risk of bloating and excess gas.

By including movement into your daily routine, even if it's just through easy exercises like yoga, stretching, or quick walks, you may significantly improve your digestive health, encourage quicker ulcer healing, and enhance your general well-being.

Managing Habits that Aggravate Ulcers

Certain behaviors can impede the healing process or exacerbate stomach ulcer symptoms. Lifestyle variables that can exacerbate ulcers include smoking, drinking alcohol, consuming large amounts of coffee, and having irregular sleep habits. Controlling these behaviors is essential for minimizing ulcer-related pain and accelerating recovery. This section examines how to change these behaviors to safeguard your stomach lining and promote digestive wellness.

Alcohol and Smoking: Minimizing Damage

1. Smoking:

Because smoking damages the stomach's protective lining and raises the production of stomach acid, it is a significant risk factor for stomach ulcers. Cigarette nicotine increases stomach acid production, which can irritate and harm the ulcer site and delay its healing. Additionally, smoking lowers blood flow to the stomach lining, which hinders the tissue's ability to heal itself.

Techniques to Lessen Damage:

- *Quit Smoking:* Giving up smoking altogether is the best strategy to stop additional harm. Seek assistance via counseling, nicotine replacement treatments, or quitting programs.

- *Minimize Nicotine Exposure:* If quitting is hard for you, start by cutting back on the amount of cigarettes you smoke each day. The damage to your stomach can still be lessened with less exposure.

2. Alcohol:

Alcohol can aggravate ulcers by irritating the stomach lining and raising stomach acid production. Additionally, heavy drinking impairs the stomach's ability to fight off dangerous bacteria and acids, which causes symptoms to worsen and healing to take longer.

Techniques to Lessen Damage:

- Limit Your Alcohol Use: Limit alcohol consumption to lessen stomach lining inflammation. Avoid alcohol entirely while the healing process is underway, if at all feasible.

- Select Non-Acidic Drinks: If you consume alcohol, choose less acidic drinks and do so sparingly. Moderation is crucial, but wine and spirits are less bothersome than beer and sugary cocktails.

Restricting Carbonated Drinks and Caffeine

Caffeine is found in coffee, tea, and many energy drinks. Consuming too much caffeine can aggravate ulcers by encouraging the stomach to create more acid. Acid reflux, which can exacerbate ulcer symptoms and delay healing, can also result from consuming too much caffeine.

Techniques for Reducing Caffeine:

- *Use Decaffeinated Options:* To lessen the effect of caffeine on your stomach, think about using decaffeinated tea or coffee. Herbal teas, such as ginger or chamomile tea, are suitable substitutes for calming the stomach.

- *Reduce Caffeine Intake Gradually:* To prevent withdrawal symptoms, reduce caffeine intake if you're accustomed to ingesting high amounts. Over time, switch to herbal teas or water instead of caffeinated beverages.

Carbonated beverages:

Sodas and sparkling water are carbonated drinks that can make you bloated and raise your stomach's pressure, resulting in pain and acid reflux. Many sodas' high sugar and acidity levels can irritate the stomach lining.

Techniques for Cutting Back on Carbonated Drinks:

Select herbal teas or still water: Water or calming herbal teas are excellent alternatives to fizzy beverages for staying hydrated without causing stomach discomfort.

Reduce Soda Consumption: If you frequently drink soda, try consuming it only on special occasions or choosing less irritating, low-acid drinks.

Digestive Health and Sleep Patterns

Poor sleep habits can negatively affect digestive health, and sleep is crucial to the healing process. In addition to impairing the body's capacity for self-healing, sleep deprivation or irregular sleep patterns can raise stress levels and stomach acid production. Furthermore, sleeping just after eating might cause acid reflux, which makes ulcers worse.

Enhancing Sleep Habits to Promote Digestive Health:

- *Create a Regular Sleep Schedule:* To maintain your body's natural rhythm, try going to bed and waking up simultaneously each day. Getting enough sleep lowers stress and promotes healing.

- *Avoid Eating Right Before Bed:* Avoid eating large meals two to three hours before bed to avoid discomfort and acid reflux. This allows your body to digest meals fully before you go to sleep.

- *Raise Your Head While You Sleep:* If you get acid reflux at night, consider raising the head of your bed by 6 to 8 inches. This position lessens discomfort by preventing stomach acid from returning to the esophagus.

Managing Stress to Improve Sleep:

Use relaxation techniques: Before bed, soothe your body and mind with relaxation methods such as deep breathing, meditation, or light stretches.

Establish a Calm Sleep Environment: To promote higher-quality sleep, keep your bedroom calm, quiet, and dark. Reducing screen time before bed can also help you fall asleep.

Support Systems and Mental Well-being

Having a chronic illness such as a stomach ulcer can be emotionally taxing and isolated. Physical discomfort, dietary limitations, and continuing medical treatments can bring on stress, anxiety, and even melancholy. To deal with these difficulties and ensure you feel heard and cared for, you must seek emotional help.

Advantages of Emotional Assistance:

Stress Reduction: Stress frequently exacerbates ulcer symptoms, and emotional support from friends, family, or support groups can lessen it.

Better Mental Health: Talking about your experiences with people who are sympathetic to your plight helps reduce anxiety and feelings of loneliness, enhancing your mental health.

Improved Coping Mechanisms: A solid support network can help you create healthy coping mechanisms by offering motivation and helpful guidance for dealing with your illness.

How to Look for Emotional Help:

Speak with those you love: Talk honestly about your feelings with your loved ones. Their empathy and support might be consoling on an emotional level.

Become a Member of a Support Group: Many people benefit from connecting with others who are experiencing similar things. Support groups can offer a secure setting for those with chronic illnesses or digestive problems to talk, learn, and get support.

Options for Therapy and Counseling

The emotional and psychological effects of having a chronic illness can occasionally be addressed with professional assistance through therapy or counseling. Managing stress, worry, or depression that may be connected to ulcer symptoms might be made more accessible by working with a therapist or counselor.

Advantages of Treatment for Ulcer Control:

- *Stress management:* Prolonged stress has a significant role in ulcer flare-ups, and treatment can assist you in learning applicable coping mechanisms.
- Cognitive behavioral therapy, or CBT, is beneficial for assisting people in altering stress-inducing negative thought patterns and behaviors, thus enhancing their mental and physical well-being.
- *Emotional Support:* Frequent therapy sessions offer a private, accepting environment where you can talk about your problems, vent your emotions, and look for answers.

Options for Therapy:

- *Personal Counseling:* Individual therapy can help you overcome emotional obstacles unique to your ulcer experience and provide you with coping mechanisms.
- Group therapy fosters community and mutual support by enabling you to talk about your experiences with others while getting expert advice.

- *Online Counseling:* Many platforms offer virtual counseling services, which provide the same advantages as traditional therapy if in-person sessions are inconvenient.

Creating a Community to Support Lifestyle Modifications

Significant lifestyle modifications, including dietary improvements, stress reduction, and habit control, are frequently necessary to manage ulcers effectively. Creating a supportive community can facilitate these adjustments and increase their long-term sustainability.

The Significance of Community Support

- *Shared Motivation:* When making challenging dietary or habit changes, having others around you who support your lifestyle can be helpful. This will help you stay accountable and inspired.

- *Encouragement and Useful Assistance:* As you adjust to new habits, friends, relatives, or neighbors can give guidance, assist with meal preparation, or offer moral support.

- *A Sense of Belonging:* Feelings of loneliness that frequently accompany chronic conditions are lessened when you are part of a group that recognizes your struggles.

How to Create a Helpful Community:

- *Make Contact with People Changing in a Similar Way:* Discover individuals who share your commitment to bettering their health, whether through local wellness initiatives, online health forums, or workout groups.

- *Engage Your Loved Ones:* Include your loved ones in your lifestyle modifications. Involving loved ones can make the process more fun, whether helping with meal preparation or engaging in stress-relieving activities.

- *Participate in Online Communities:* Numerous websites provide communities devoted to general well-being, digestive health, or ulcer management. You can interact with others in these areas, exchange advice, ask questions, and support one another.

Integrating Ulcer Management into Daily Life

In addition to dietary modifications, managing stomach ulcers requires lifestyle modifications incorporated into your everyday activities. By quickly incorporating these adjustments into your daily routine, ulcer management will feel less taxing and more long-lasting. This section looks at managing your ulcers while establishing habits, organizing meals, and overcoming obstacles like eating out or traveling.

Establishing a Successful Routine

Creating a daily habit that promotes ulcer healing is the secret to long-term success. Dietary, stress-reduction, and exercise consistency all aid in controlling stomach acid formation, averting flare-ups, and accelerating the healing process.

How to Establish a Routine:

- *Establish Regular Meal Schedules:* Overeating can cause excessive acid production, so eating short, balanced meals simultaneously daily helps normalize digestion. Try to have five or six short meals throughout the day, with no extended intervals in between.

- *Include Relaxation Techniques:* Set aside a short period each day for stress-relieving exercises like yoga, deep breathing, or mindfulness. Reducing stress facilitates improved digestion by lowering the formation of stomach acid.

- *Plan a Gentle Workout:* Frequent low-impact exercise, such as yoga, swimming, or walking, can help lower stress and enhance digestion. Include exercise in your daily schedule; try to get it in 20 to 30 minutes on most days.

The Significance of Routine

- *Cuts Down on Uncertainties:* You may follow your ulcer treatment plan without worrying about what to eat or how to handle stress when you have a routine since it lessens decision fatigue.

- *Encourages Healing:* Maintaining a consistent diet and way of life helps the body heal, avoid flare-ups, and maintain long-term digestive health.

Planning and Preparing Meals for Busy Lives

Maintaining an ulcer-friendly diet can be difficult when you have a busy schedule, but meal planning and preparation can help ensure you always have wholesome, calming foods. By planning your meals ahead of time, you can lessen the temptation to reach for convenience foods that could aggravate your ulcer.

Advice on Planning and Preparing Meals:

- *Prepare meals in large quantities:* Schedule time weekly to prepare large amounts of meals, including grilled chicken with veggies, soups, and stews. Store quick and simple meals in portioned containers throughout the week.

- *Stock Up on Ulcer-Friendly Staples:* Keep simple, calming meals like oatmeal, yogurt, bananas, lean meats, and vegetables in your cupboard and refrigerator. This guarantees that solutions are always available that won't upset your stomach.

- *Utilize a Weekly Meal Schedule:* Make a weekly food plan emphasizing wholesome, easy recipes. This guarantees that your meals will assist in treating your ulcers and lessen the stress associated with choosing what to eat each day.

- *Snack Prep:* To ensure you always have a nutritious snack to reach for in between meals, prepare ulcer-friendly foods like yogurt, chopped fruit, or whole-grain crackers in advance.

Organizing Meals for Busy Days:

- *Fast breakfasts:* Make smoothies or overnight oats the night before for a quick and calming start to the day.

- Simple, easily digestible lunches, such as a turkey wrap with soft veggies or a quinoa salad with grilled chicken, should be packed the night before.

- *Easy Dinners:* Prepare meals to reheat or make fast stir-fries with vegetables and lean proteins if you're pressed for time in the evening.

Advice for Patients with Ulcers on Traveling and Eating Out

For people with stomach ulcers, eating out or traveling can be difficult because they frequently have less control over what they consume. Nevertheless, if they plan and make thoughtful decisions, they can still have these experiences without jeopardizing their ulcer treatment.

- *Travel Advice for Ulcer Patients:* Bring Snacks: To avoid eating unhealthful or irritating meals at airports or petrol stations, bring ulcer-friendly snacks like bananas, rice cakes, yogurt, or whole-grain crackers.

- *Keep Yourself Hydrated:* Avoid carbonated or caffeinated drinks, which might upset your stomach, and drink lots of water during your trip.

- *Investigate Your Destination:* If you're visiting a new location, look for local eateries or supermarkets that provide calming, healthful options. Choose eateries that offer grilled, steamed, or essential dishes.

Tips for Eating Out:

- *Pick Restaurants Carefully:* Seek out eateries that serve various healthful dishes, like whole grains, grilled meats, and steamed veggies. Avoid restaurants that serve fatty or spicy meals or quick food.

- *Ask for Changes:* Don't hesitate to ask the waiter to change your order. You can also request your food made without a lot of fats, spices, or sauces or grilled or steam-cooked.

- *Portion Control:* Large amounts at restaurants might be uncomfortable. To prevent overindulging, consider splitting a meal or packing half to leave.

- *Choose Calm Drinks:* When ordering drinks, choose low-acid alternatives, herbal teas (such as ginger or chamomile), or water. Avoid coffee, alcohol, and fizzy beverages.

- *Plan Ahead:* If you are sure you will be eating out, look for ulcer-friendly options on the restaurant's internet menu in advance. This lessens the pressure of having to make snap decisions while eating.

Foods That Are Travel-Friendly:

- *Packets of oatmeal:* Oatmeal is a healthy and satisfying alternative to bread when traveling. It is simple to make with hot water.

- Rice cakes or plain crackers are portable, light, and easily digested snacks.

- *Soft Fruits:* Applesauce or bananas make excellent, stomach-friendly travel companions.

- *Turkey or Grilled Chicken Wraps:* Lean protein and tender veggies combine to provide a convenient travel lunch.

Monitoring Your Health

Managing stomach ulcers and avoiding complications requires constant health monitoring. Maintaining long-term digestive health requires routine exams, early detection of flare-ups, and modification of your treatment plan as needed.

By remaining alert and proactive, you can identify issues early and modify your lifestyle or course of medication to encourage healing and stop ulcers from returning.

Routine Examinations and Screenings

Routine medical examinations and screenings are essential to track the effectiveness of your ulcer treatment and ensure no new issues develop. Even when symptoms subside, it's crucial to see your doctor regularly to ensure the ulcer has completely healed and to look for any underlying problems that could raise the chance of recurrence.

Advantages of Frequent Exams:

- *Monitor the Healing Process:* During follow-up visits, your doctor can evaluate the healing of your ulcer and determine whether your treatment plan needs to be modified.

- *Keep an eye out for any complications:* Complications like bleeding, perforation, or infection can occasionally result from ulcers. Endoscopies and other routine tests aid in identifying these problems early on before they worsen.

- *Address Additional Digestive Issues:* Exams also offer a chance to address any additional digestive health issues that may impact your general health, such as gastritis or acid reflux.

Suggested Screenings:

Endoscope: Your doctor can suggest a follow-up endoscope to check the stomach lining and ensure the ulcer has completely healed. This test is especially crucial if your symptoms develop or continue.

H. pylori Testing: If an H. pylori infection caused your ulcer, your doctor may perform a blood, stool, or breath test to ensure the disease has been eliminated.

Understanding the Signs of Flare-Ups

Ulcers can occasionally recur even after they have first healed. To stop the problem from getting worse, it's critical to recognize the early warning symptoms of a flare-up. Early symptom detection allows you to take action to treat the issue before it causes more problems.

Typical signs of flare-ups include:

- *Burning or Gnawing Pain:* A persistent burning feeling in the upper abdomen, particularly at night or between meals, could indicate worsening your ulcer.

- *Bloating or Nausea:* After eating, persistent bloating, indigestion, or nausea may indicate your ulcer is reoccurring.

- *Acid Reflux or Heartburn:* If you frequently get acid reflux or heartburn, especially after eating, this may indicate that your ulcer is flared up.

- Changes in appetite or unexplained weight loss should be considered seriously as possible indicators of ulcer recurrence, especially if they are accompanied by post-meal discomfort.

How to Respond When Symptoms Are Noticed:

- *Take Action Now:* Do not postpone therapy if you observe any indications of a flare-up. If you experience new or reoccurring symptoms, speak with your healthcare professional.

- *Examine Your Lifestyle and Diet:* Stress, food, and other lifestyle choices might cause a flare-up. Examine your diet and any recent dietary adjustments to determine possible explanations.

- *Modify Medication:* If symptoms return, your doctor may need to change your prescriptions. For example, they may need to increase proton pump inhibitors (PPIs) or resume H. pylori drugs.

Modifying Treatment Programs as Necessary

Your treatment plan should adapt as your condition does. Your treatment approach should be adaptable enough to consider new developments because stomach ulcers might react differently. Collaborating closely with your physician can modify your treatment to guarantee continued healing and avoid recurrences.

When to Modify Your Therapy Strategy:

- *Symptoms that are persistent or getting worse:* It can be essential to change prescriptions, up dosages, or look into other therapies if your symptoms don't go away even after you've followed your treatment plan.

- *New difficulties:* Your treatment plan will need to be adjusted to handle any new challenges that may occur, such as bleeding, infection, or excruciating pain. More extensive medical procedures like surgery or more diagnostic testing can be required.

- *Ineffective Drugs:* Some drugs may become ineffective over time, or their adverse effects may become unbearable. In such situations, your doctor might suggest other therapies, including lifestyle changes, or change your prescription.

Work Together with Your Physician:

- *Regular Interaction:* Maintain constant contact with your healthcare physician, particularly if your situation changes. Regular updates allow your doctor to make well-informed judgments about modifying your treatment strategy.

- *Examine Lifestyle Modifications:* If lifestyle factors like diet, stress, or exercise are causing persistent symptoms, you might need to review your lifestyle modifications to promote improved ulcer management.

NOTES:

CHAPTER FOUR: Cooking Techniques for Ulcer-Friendly Meals

When dealing with stomach ulcers, what you eat is equally important as how you prepare your meals. This chapter will examine cooking techniques and ingredient selections that help heal ulcers while making your meals nutritious and pleasurable. The emphasis will be on stomach-friendly cooking methods, using ingredients that promote healing, and creating delectable dishes without exacerbating your problems.

We'll start by discussing safe cooking techniques, including steaming, boiling, baking, and avoiding deep-frying and heavy seasonings. Next, we'll look at choosing nutrients that promote gut health, such as fresh, whole foods over processed ones, whole grains, lean meats, and omega-3-rich foods.

Seasoning is essential for generating tasty dishes that won't irritate your stomach. You'll learn how to utilize delectable but gentle flavors, such as herbs and spices, that promote digestion while avoiding substances that can cause discomfort. In addition, we'll go over meal preparation strategies that make your food more digestible and advise you on portioning and timing your meals to reduce aggravation.

Finally, this chapter will include budget-friendly recipes that promote healing. It will emphasize low-cost, ulcer-friendly foods and tactics such as batch cooking to help you save time while staying healthy. Whether cooking for yourself or your family, these approaches will help you create relaxing, fulfilling meals that improve digestive health.

Safe Cooking Techniques for Ulcers

Cooking skills are essential in managing stomach ulcers since particular methods can soothe or irritate the lining. To improve healing, it is critical to utilize approaches that limit fat content, avoid irritating spices, and keep the nutritional worth of ingredients without causing excessive acid production.

Steaming, boiling, and baking.

These gentle cooking methods are great for ulcer patients because they preserve the food's natural nutrients without adding excess fat or harsh seasonings that may irritate the stomach.

- Steaming is an excellent method for preserving nutrients in vegetables, seafood, and lean meats while keeping the food soft and straightforward to digest.

- **Boiling:** Ideal for cereals, veggies, and lean proteins, boiling keeps the food wet and easy on the stomach.

- Baking without extra fats can be an excellent method for cooking meats and veggies. Use parchment paper or foil to seal in moisture and keep the meal soft.

Avoiding Deep-frying and Spicy Seasonings

Deep-fried foods are high in fat and can cause excessive stomach acid production, resulting in irritation. Furthermore, hot seasonings such as chile, black pepper, and heavy sauces should be avoided because they might irritate the stomach lining and worsen ulcer symptoms.

- **Avoid Deep-Frying:** Instead of frying, try baking or grilling with minimal oil. This lowers fat levels while keeping meals light and ulcer-friendly.

- **Limit Spicy Seasonings:** Instead of hot spices, use mild herbs and non-irritating flavors like ginger, turmeric, or garlic to provide flavor without causing pain.

Cooking with Healthy Oils and Fats.

Using the correct fats is critical for producing ulcer-friendly meals. Healthy fats like olive and avocado are more easily digestible and cause less irritation than heavier oils or butter.

Use olive or avocado oil: These oils are heart-healthy and low in saturated fat, making them easy on the stomach. Use them carefully while sautéing or roasting meals.

Avoid heavy oils and butter. Limit your usage of butter or lard, which can raise fat levels and cause excessive acid production, exacerbating ulcer symptoms.

Choosing Ingredients that Support Healing

Choosing the proper nutrients is critical for treating ulcers and boosting healing. Fresh, unprocessed, nutrient-dense ingredients help to nourish the stomach lining, reduce inflammation, and give the nutrients required for recovery. This section discusses how eating fresh foods over processed foods, including whole grains and legumes, and consuming lean proteins and omega-3-rich foods can help heal ulcers.

Fresh Versus Processed Ingredients

Fresh foods are high in essential nutrients, free of additives, and gentler on the digestive system. On the other hand, processed meals frequently contain preservatives, high sodium levels, unhealthy fats, and artificial tastes, all of which can worsen ulcers and disrupt the healing process.

- *Fresh ingredients:* Choose veggies, fruits, whole grains, and lean proteins. These meals contain vitamins, fiber, and antioxidants, which help to heal and reduce inflammation.

- *Processed Ingredients:* Processed foods with high salt and fat content, such as canned soups, packaged snacks, and frozen dinners, might irritate the stomach. They also lack the essential minerals required for repair; thus, it is recommended that their intake be limited.

Incorporating whole grains and legumes

Whole grains and legumes are high in fiber, which assists digestion and lowers stomach acid levels. These foods provide sustained energy and promote intestinal health without creating inflammation.

- Whole grains, including brown rice, oats, quinoa, and whole wheat, are great options. The fiber in these grains aids digestion, reduces bloating, and promotes a healthy gut microbiota.

- Legumes: Beans, lentils, and chickpeas are abundant in protein and fiber, making them excellent plant-based ulcer treatments. However, for some sensitive to legumes, soaking them before cooking can make them simpler to stomach.

Lean Proteins and Omega-3-Rich Foods

Lean proteins and omega-3 fatty acids help reduce inflammation and promote the healing of stomach ulcers. These proteins are easily digestible and include necessary amino acids to heal the stomach lining.

- *Lean Proteins:* Include lean meats like chicken, turkey, and fish, as well as plant-based proteins like tofu and tempeh. Unlike fatty portions of meat, these proteins are less prone to cause increased stomach acid production.

- *Omega-3 Rich Foods:* Fatty fish such as salmon, mackerel, and sardines contain omega-3s, which have anti-inflammatory characteristics that can calm and mend the stomach lining. Plant-based choices include chia seeds, flaxseeds, and walnuts, all high in omega-3 fatty acids.

- Choose fresh, unprocessed products and incorporate whole grains, legumes, lean meats, and omega-3-rich foods to produce a nutrient-dense diet that promotes ulcer healing, inflammation reduction, and long-term digestive health.

Flavorful but Gentle Seasoning Options

One of the most important things to do when managing stomach ulcers is to season your meals with attention. Some spices and seasonings can worsen ulcers by increasing the amount of stomach acid or irritating the lining. On the other hand, other spices and seasonings can improve flavor while helping digestion and healing. You can enjoy delectable meals without experiencing discomfort if you select calming herbs and spices and steer clear of those that induce inflammation.

Herbs and Spices that Aid Digestion (Turmeric, Ginger)

In addition to imparting flavor, particular herbs and spices aid digestion and contribute to the reduction of inflammation. These components are accessible on the stomach and can be incorporated into meals suitable for people who suffer from ulcers.

Turmeric: Known for its anti-inflammatory effects, turmeric is a strong spice that helps soothe the stomach lining. Curcumin in this product has been demonstrated to reduce inflammation and aid the healing of ulcers.

Ginger: Ginger is generally renowned for its digestive properties. It helps alleviate nausea, relaxes the stomach, and aids with digestion. Ginger can be used in teas, soups, and stir-fries for a relaxing flavor.

Other Soothing Herbs: Basil, parsley, dill, and cilantro are mild herbs that improve flavor without upsetting the stomach. These herbs are ideal for seasoning salads, soups, and sauces.

Avoiding Irritating Seasonings (Chili, Black Pepper)

Certain spices and seasonings can worsen ulcers by boosting stomach acid production or irritating the lining. It's recommended to avoid these if you have a sensitive stomach or are in the process of mending an ulcer.

Chili Peppers: Spicy seasonings like chili powder, cayenne pepper, and spicy sauces can irritate the stomach lining and worsen ulcer symptoms. These should be avoided or significantly reduced.

Black Pepper: While a ubiquitous condiment, black pepper can accelerate acid production and cause discomfort in particular persons with ulcers. It's better to substitute it with milder alternatives like fresh herbs.

Acidic and Strong Spices: Mustard, horseradish, and vinegar can also increase acid production and worsen ulcer symptoms. Thus, they should be limited.

Using Citrus Alternatives for Flavor

Citrus fruits like lemons, limes, and oranges are widely used in flavor recipes but can be excessively acidic for persons with ulcers. However, there are various ways to liven up meals without creating irritation.

Light Vinegar (in moderation): While more pungent vinegar should be avoided, light choices like apple cider vinegar (in small amounts) can be used for flavoring, though monitoring tolerance is crucial.

Herbs for Brightness: Herbs like lemongrass or lemon balm can impart a zesty flavor without the acidity of lemons. They can be used in marinades, sauces, and teas.

Low-Acid Fruits: If you want to add a bit of sweetness or tanginess, choose lower-acid fruits such as apples, pears, or melons. These fruits are mild on the stomach while offering flavor.

Preparing Meals for Easy Digestion

Preparing meals that encourage simple digestion is vital when controlling stomach ulcers. Softer foods and particular cooking procedures minimize the load on your digestive system, helping prevent discomfort and inflammation. By softening foods, pureeing or mashing, and cooking meals in advance, you may ensure that your diet is pleasant on the stomach and aids the healing process.

Softening Foods for Gentle Digestion

Softening foods makes them easier to digest and lowers the danger of irritating the stomach lining. This can be especially crucial for ulcer patients since hard foods can cause bloating or irritation.

Cooking Methods: Steaming, boiling, and simmering are terrific ways to soften vegetables, cereals, and meats without adding extra fat or harsh flavors. These processes make the meal delicate, guaranteeing it is easy on your stomach.

Choose Soft Fruits and Vegetables: Opt for soft, easy-to-digest fruits like bananas, applesauce, or pears and cooked vegetables such as carrots, squash, and sweet potatoes. Cooking these items makes them even more digestible.

Soak Grains and Legumes: If you consume grains like oats or legumes such as beans and lentils, consider soaking them before cooking. This softens their texture and makes them more digestible, helping relieve gas and bloating.

Pureeing and Mashing Techniques

For those with more sensitive stomachs, pureeing or mashing food might make it even simpler to digest. These procedures break down the food into smaller, softer particles that are friendlier on the stomach lining and less likely to irritate.

Pureeing: Use a blender or food processor to puree soups, vegetables, and fruits. Smooth, pureed foods are easier to digest and help minimize discomfort. For example, a blended vegetable soup made with vegetables like carrots, squash, and potatoes can be calming and nourishing.

Mashing: Mashing foods such as potatoes, sweet potatoes, and bananas is another excellent approach to generating soft, readily digestible meals. Mashed foods are pleasant and require less effort to chew, lessening the stress on the stomach.

Soups and Smoothies: Soups and smoothies made from pureed vegetables or fruits are fantastic solutions for ulcer patients. They deliver necessary nutrients while being easy on the digestive tract.

Prepping Meals Ahead of Time

Preparing meals in advance ensures that you always have ulcer-friendly foods, making it more straightforward to stick to a soothing diet, even on hectic days. It also lets you focus on cooking using gentle techniques and ingredients, eliminating the temptation to eat manufactured or irritating dishes.

Batch Cooking: Prepare large servings of soft foods, soups, or mashed dishes that may be kept and reheated throughout the week. This helps guarantee you always have an ulcer-friendly meal ready to go.

Freezing Meals: Freeze individual amounts of pureed soups, cooked grains, or steamed vegetables. Freezing meals beforehand ensures you have nutritional options even when you're short on time.

Snack Prep: Prepare soft, easy-to-digest snacks in advance, such as applesauce, yogurt, or mashed bananas. Keeping snacks on hand helps you avoid unhealthy or unpleasant dietary choices.

Best Practices for Portioning and Timing

Proper portioning and timing of meals are crucial for treating ulcers and decreasing stomach inflammation. Eating smaller, more frequent meals helps manage acid production, while avoiding large portions and late-night eating can reduce discomfort and encourage recovery. This section discusses the best practices for regulating meal quantities and scheduling to improve digestive health.

Small, Frequent Meals for Less Irritation

Eating smaller, frequent meals daily can help minimize stomach irritation and prevent excessive acid production. Large meals can overload the stomach and produce discomfort, whereas smaller servings are more accessible to digest and less likely to develop ulcer symptoms.

Benefits: Small, frequent meals prevent the stomach from growing excessively full, which can create pressure and acid reflux. Maintaining constant digestion can minimize spikes in acid production that may irritate ulcers.

How to Implement: Aim to eat five to six small meals a day instead of the typical three large ones. For example, consider a light snack between breakfast and lunch and another between lunch and supper, ensuring that each meal is balanced and ulcer-friendly.

Avoiding Late-Night Eating

Eating late at night can raise the risk of acid reflux and indigestion, both of which can worsen ulcer symptoms. When you lie down soon after eating, stomach acid is more likely to flow back into the esophagus, resulting in discomfort and irritation.

Why It Matters: Late-night meals can disrupt digestion and create symptoms like acid reflux, especially if you consume large or heavy meals before bedtime. This can worsen ulcers and impede recovery.

Best Practices: Finish your last meal or snack at least 2-3 hours before bed. This gives your body adequate time to digest meals before lying down, lowering the danger of reflux or pain. Opt for a light dinner that's easy to digest, such as grilled salmon and steamed veggies.

Portion Control for Ulcer-Friendly Meals

Portion control is vital for avoiding overloading the stomach with large quantities of food, which can boost acid production. Keeping quantities reasonable helps control digestion and lowers the likelihood of bloating or discomfort.

Why Portion Control is Important: Large amounts can cause the stomach to stretch, resulting in increased acid production and pressure on the stomach lining. This might worsen ulcers and create discomfort.

How to Control Portions:

Use Smaller Plates: Using smaller plates helps you regulate portion sizes visually and lowers the urge to overeat.

Balance Nutrients: Ensure each meal includes a balance of lean proteins, fiber-rich grains, and mild veggies. Avoid heaping your plate with heavy, greasy, or spicy foods that may irritate the stomach.

Listen to Your Body: Eat gently and quit when you feel unsatisfied. This helps prevent overeating and lessens the strain on your stomach.

Budget-Friendly Ulcer Recipes

Managing stomach ulcers with a healthy diet doesn't have to be expensive. By picking economical products, making meals in batches, and focusing on essential, nutritional recipes, you may assist your ulcer healing while staying on a budget. This section covers cost-effective approaches to maintaining an ulcer-friendly diet that promotes healing and decreases inflammation.

Affordable Ingredients that Heal

Numerous inexpensive, ulcer-friendly foods can be incorporated into your everyday meals. These foods are mild on the stomach, full of nutrients, and easy to include in basic meals.

Oats: Oatmeal is a relaxing, fiber-rich breakfast option that helps lower acid production and promotes digestion. It's inexpensive and may be bought in quantity for long-term use.

Bananas: A terrific budget-friendly fruit, bananas are easy on the stomach and give critical nutrients like potassium and fiber. They can be eaten alone or added to smoothies, porridge, or yogurt.

Brown Rice and Quinoa: Both brown rice and quinoa are affordable whole grains that promote healthy digestion. They give fiber and energy without causing discomfort, making them the perfect meal.

Canned Beans and Lentils: Beans and lentils are budget-friendly, high in protein and fiber, and easy to digest when prepared properly. They're flexible and can be used in soups, salads, and stews.

Sweet Potatoes: Sweet potatoes are a mild, nutrient-dense alternative that may be baked, mashed, or added to stews. They are rich in fiber, vitamins, and antioxidants, making them suitable for intestinal health.

Batch Cooking for the Week

Batch cooking helps save both time and money while ensuring you always have ulcer-friendly foods on hand. By cooking significant portions of meals in advance, you may freeze or refrigerate them throughout the week, making it more straightforward to stick to a balanced diet, even on hectic days.

Benefits of Batch Cooking:

- ✓ Saves time during the week, minimizing the daily need to cook.
- ✓ Ensures you always have nutritional, ulcer-friendly meals ready to consume.
- ✓ Helps prevent the urge to rely on processed or quick foods that may aggravate ulcers.

Batch Cooking Ideas:

Soups and Stews: Prepare a large pot of vegetable or chicken soup using carrots, zucchini, brown rice, and lean proteins. Store in sections for quick reheating.

Cooked Grains: Make a large amount of brown rice, quinoa, or oats that can be used as a base for several meals throughout the week.

Roasted veggies: Roast veggies (sweet potatoes, carrots, squash) in abundance and store them in the fridge to add to meals.

Simple, Nutritious Recipes on a Budget

Here are a few simple and budget-friendly ulcer-friendly dishes that are both nutritious and quick to make:

1. Oatmeal with Banana and Honey

INGREDIENTS:

- 1 cup oats
- one banana (sliced)
- one tablespoon of honey
- 2 cups water or almond milk

INSTRUCTIONS: Cook the oats in water or almond milk until tender.

Top with banana slices and drizzle with honey for a calming, easy-to-digest breakfast.

2. Vegetable and Lentil Soup

INGREDIENTS:

- 1 cup red lentils (rinsed)
- one carrot (chopped)
- one zucchini (chopped)
- one sweet potato (chopped)
- 4 cups vegetable broth

INSTRUCTIONS:

- In a big pot, combine all ingredients and boil.
- Reduce heat and simmer for 30-40 minutes until vegetables and lentils are cooked.
- Season with mild herbs like parsley or turmeric for extra flavor.

3. *Baked Sweet Potatoes with Avocado*

INGREDIENTS:

- two sweet potatoes
- one avocado (mashed)
- Olive oil
- Salt and pepper (optional)

INSTRUCTIONS:

- Preheat the oven to 400°F (200°C). Pierce the sweet potatoes with a fork and bake for 45-60 minutes until soft.
- Slice the sweet potatoes and top with mashed avocado and olive oil.

4. Brown Rice and Bean Salad

INGREDIENTS:

- 1 cup cooked brown rice
- one can of black beans (drained and rinsed)
- 1/2 cucumber (chopped) 1 tablespoon olive oil
- Fresh parsley or cilantro

INSTRUCTIONS: Combine the cooked brown rice, beans, and cucumber in a bowl.

Drizzle with olive oil and toss with herbs for a refreshing, protein-packed dinner.

CHAPTER FIVE: Medications and Natural Remedies

Medication and natural remedies play critical roles in managing stomach ulcers. Whether an H. pylori infection, excessive stomach acid, or prolonged use of NSAIDs causes your ulcer, treatment often includes a combination of medications to reduce symptoms, promote healing, and address the underlying causes. In addition to medicines, natural remedies, and supplements, they can support gut health, ulcer healing, and drugs.

This chapter will guide you through both medical treatments and natural remedies, helping you understand how these methods can complement each other. We'll start by discussing common medications recommended for ulcers, such as proton pump inhibitors (PPIs), H2 blockers, and antibiotics for H. pylori. These medications reduce acid production, support healing, and address infections.

Next, we'll study natural supplements and remedies like probiotics, licorice root, and slippery elm. These natural choices can support digestion and provide additional relief when combined with medical treatments.

We'll also discuss integrating medications with dietary changes, focusing on timing medicines with meals, avoiding potential irritation, and monitoring for side effects. This will help ensure your treatment plan works smoothly with your diet and lifestyle.

Additionally, we'll cover the possible side effects of medications, such as allergic reactions and digestive issues. Understanding these side effects can help you stay proactive and alert your healthcare provider if any problems appear.

Finally, we'll consider combining medical treatment with alternative therapies, including acupuncture, massage, and herbal medicine, to offer a holistic approach to ulcer care. To maximize the benefits, you'll learn to mix these therapies safely with your prescribed treatments.

This chapter will thoroughly examine balancing medications, natural remedies, and alternative treatments to manage and heal stomach ulcers effectively.

Common Medications for Ulcer Treatment

Stomach ulcers frequently require medical attention to facilitate healing and alleviate symptoms such as pain and discomfort. Medications are commonly used to lower stomach acid, protect the stomach lining, and, if necessary, treat bacterial diseases such as Helicobacter pylori. Proton pump inhibitors (PPIs), H2 blockers and antibiotics, and antibiotics for H. pylori are the three primary types of ulcer treatments.

Proton pump inhibitors (PPIs)

Proton Pump Inhibitors (PPIs) are among the most widely given drugs for treating stomach ulcers. They act by inhibiting the enzyme in the stomach lining that produces stomach acid. PPIs inhibit acid production, allowing ulcers to heal more effectively and alleviating pain and acid reflux symptoms.

Common PPIs include;

Omeprazole (Prilosec), Lansoprazole (Prevacid), esomeprazole (Nexium), and pantoprazole (Protonix).

How PPIs Help

- Reduced acid production: Lowering stomach acid levels prevents further discomfort and allows the ulcer to heal.
- Less acid in the stomach fosters a healing environment and reduces ulcer size.

- Relieves symptoms: PPIs alleviate symptoms such as burning pain, acid reflux, and indigestion, which improves the quality of life during recovery.

- PPIs are typically taken once or twice daily and, when used as directed, are effective in treating most ulcers.

H2 blockers and antacids

H2 blockers are another type of drug that reduces stomach acid production, but they function differently than PPIs. Instead of inhibiting the acid-producing enzyme, H2 blockers keep histamine from triggering acid formation in the stomach.

Common H2 blockers include

Ranitidine (Zantac) was recalled due to contamination concerns, Famotidine (Pepcid) and Cimetidine (Tagamet),

H2 blockers can alleviate ulcer symptoms and promote the healing of the stomach lining by lowering acid levels. However, they are less effective than PPIs.

- Antacids are over-the-counter drugs that neutralize stomach acid and temporarily relieve symptoms such as heartburn and indigestion. They do not reduce acid production but provide brief comfort by neutralizing the acid in the stomach.

Common antacids include

- Calcium Carbonate (Tums).
- Magnesium Hydroxide (Magnesia Milk)
- Aluminum hydroxide (Maalox)

How H2 Blockers and Antacids Work:

- **H2 Blockers:** Reduce acid production in the stomach, allowing ulcers to heal and alleviating symptoms such as burning pain.

- **Antacids:** Provide immediate relief from acid-related symptoms; however, their effects are temporary and should be used in conjunction with other drugs for long-term healing.

Antibiotics against H. pylori

Antibiotics are essential to remove Helicobacter pylori (H. pylori), which is the bacteria that causes ulcers. Treating the bacterial infection is critical for healing the ulcer and preventing new ulcers from forming.

Common Antibiotics for H. Pylori:

- Amoxicillin
- Clarithromycin
- Metronidazole
- Tetracycline

These antibiotics are frequently administered as part of a triple therapy regimen consisting of two antibiotics and a PPI to eradicate bacteria while reducing stomach acid.

How Antibiotics Help

- Eliminate H. pylori Infection: By removing the bacteria, antibiotics treat the underlying cause of the ulcer and allow the stomach lining to heal.
- Prevent Ulcer recurrence: Successful treatment of the H. pylori infection lowers the risk of subsequent ulcers.
- Antibiotic treatment typically lasts 10-14 days, and it is critical to finish the entire course to eliminate the bacteria.

Natural Supplements and Remedies

In addition to traditional pharmaceuticals, many patients with stomach ulcers find comfort in natural nutrients and therapies that enhance gut health, reduce inflammation, and encourage healing. Natural therapies can supplement medical treatments, providing additional assistance while avoiding the unpleasant side effects of some drugs. In this part, we look at how probiotics, licorice root (DGL), slippery elm, and marshmallow root can help manage ulcers.

Probiotics and Gut Health

Probiotics are good bacteria that contribute to a healthy balance of microorganisms in the gut, which is essential for digestive health. Probiotics can also help heal ulcers by restoring the gut's normal flora, which is mainly caused by Helicobacter pylori infections.

Advantages of Probiotics for Ulcer Management:

- *Supports Gut Flora:* Probiotics help replace beneficial bacteria in the gut, especially after taking antibiotics for H. pylori infections, which can upset the microbiome.

- *Reduces Inflammation:* Some probiotic strains have anti-inflammatory qualities that help soothe the stomach lining and aid in healing.

- *Combats H. pylori:* Some research suggests that probiotics may limit H. pylori growth, lowering its influence on the stomach lining and improving antibiotic efficacy.

Probiotic-Rich Foods and Supplements:

Live cultures in yogurt, kefir, sauerkraut, and kimchi

Probiotic supplements (with strains like Lactobacillus and Bifidobacterium)

Probiotics can help maintain intestinal balance, reduce inflammation, and heal ulcers.

Licorice Root and Deglycorrhizinated Licorice (DGL)

Licorice root has traditionally been used as a natural treatment for digestive problems like ulcers. However, because ordinary licorice includes glycyrrhizin, which can produce adverse effects such as elevated blood pressure, Deglycyrrhizinated Licorice (DGL) is widely used to cure ulcers. DGL is a type of licorice that has had its glycyrrhizin eliminated, making it safe for long-term consumption.

Advantages of DGL for Ulcer Healing:

- Increases Mucus formation: DGL stimulates mucus formation in the stomach lining, which forms a protective barrier against stomach acid and allows the ulcer to heal.
- Licorice root has anti-inflammatory qualities that can calm the stomach lining and relieve discomfort.
- DGL promotes healing by boosting protective mucus and lowering acid irritation to the stomach lining.

How To Use DGL:

- DGL is available in chewable tablets and powder form and should be taken 15-30 minutes before meals. Chewing the tablet promotes the development of protective mucus in the stomach.
- DGL is a natural choice for ulcer management. It can be safely taken with other treatments to alleviate symptoms and aid healing.

Slippery Elm, Marshmallow Root

Slippery elm and marshmallow root are soothing herbal treatments often used to treat digestive ailments like ulcers. These herbs create a protective layer on the stomach lining, minimizing discomfort and boosting recovery.

- Slippery elm includes mucilage, which protects the stomach and esophagus lining from acid and discomfort.
- Slippery elm promotes healing by forming a protective barrier that allows ulcers to heal while relieving symptoms such as pain and discomfort.
- Reduces Inflammation: Its anti-inflammatory effects aid in alleviating swelling and discomfort in the digestive tract.
- Marshmallow root includes mucilage, which forms a protective layer over the stomach lining and soothes inflammation from acid.
- Promotes Digestive Health: It reduces inflammation and soothes the digestive tract, effectively treating stomach ulcers and other inflammatory diseases.
- Slippery elm and marshmallow root can be consumed in various forms, including teas, capsules, and powders. Drinking tea made from these herbs before meals can help relieve symptoms by covering the stomach lining and reducing irritation from food or acid.

Integrating Medications with Dietary Changes

Combining your medications with suitable dietary adjustments is critical to guarantee maximum effectiveness and reduce adverse effects when treating stomach ulcers. Successful ulcer treatment requires proper drug timing, avoidance of foods that may irritate the stomach lining, and monitoring for potential adverse effects. Coordinating your food with your pharmaceutical regimen can speed healing and lessen discomfort.

Coordinating Medications with Meals

The timing of your drugs about meals influences their efficacy and stomach tolerance. Some medications, such as proton pump inhibitors (PPIs), are most effective before meals, while others, such as antacids, may be more beneficial after meals.

Best Practices For Timing Medications:

- *Proton Pump Inhibitors (PPI):* Medications like omeprazole and lansoprazole work best when given 30 to 60 minutes before a meal, often breakfast. This allows them to lower stomach acid levels before eating.

- *Antacids:* These are usually given after meals or when symptoms appear to neutralize stomach acid. If you take both PPIs and antacids, space them out so they don't interfere.

- Antibiotics for H. pylori should be given with food to avoid stomach irritation or nausea. Follow your doctor's timing guidelines for the best outcomes.

By adequately scheduling your prescriptions with meals, you may guarantee that they work and limit the chance of stomach distress.

Preventing Medication-Related Irritations

Certain medications, particularly antibiotics and anti-inflammatory drugs, might irritate the stomach lining, causing discomfort or exacerbating ulcer symptoms. To reduce this discomfort, avoid particular foods and follow dietary practices that complement your prescription plan.

Tips for avoiding irritation:

Avoid spicy, acidic, or fatty foods. These meals can irritate the stomach lining, especially while taking antibiotics or NSAIDs. Eat bland, mild foods like steamed vegetables, lean meats, and whole grains.

Eat Soft, Easily Digestible Foods: Soft foods like oatmeal, bananas, and cooked vegetables are gentler on the stomach and can help protect the lining from irritation caused by drugs.

Stay Hydrated. Drinking plenty of water helps drain toxins and ensures drugs travel through your digestive system without irritating it.

Use Probiotics: If you're taking antibiotics to treat H. pylori, incorporating probiotics into your diet will help replace beneficial bacteria in your gut and lower the chance of digestive side effects like diarrhea.

Taking these precautions can help reduce the irritation that some drugs may cause and promote better digestion during treatment.

Monitoring Side Effects.

Monitoring potential side effects when using ulcer treatments is critical. Some drugs, including antibiotics, PPIs and H2 blockers can cause gastrointestinal symptoms such as nausea, diarrhea, and constipation. Awareness of these side effects and addressing them early can help avoid difficulties.

Common side effects of antibiotics, especially those used to treat H. pylori, include nausea and stomach upset. Eating small, regular meals and avoiding heavy or oily foods can help to alleviate nausea.

Diarrhea or Constipation: PPIs and antibiotics might cause changes in bowel habits. To maintain regular bowel movements, ensure you consume adequate fiber and keep hydrated.

Acid Rebound: Stopping PPIs abruptly can result in a rebound rise in stomach acid production, exacerbating symptoms. Always with your doctor before changing your medication.

- **Severe or Persistent Side Effects:** If you have severe side effects, such as persistent nausea, vomiting, or severe diarrhea, call your doctor immediately.

- **Allergic Reactions:** Symptoms of an allergic reaction include redness, trouble breathing, and swelling. If any of these symptoms appear, get medical attention.

- Regular check-ins with your healthcare practitioner and monitoring how your body responds to drugs can allow you to adapt your treatment plan and manage any side effects as soon as possible.

Integrating drugs with dietary modifications entails carefully timing your medications with meals, selecting foods that reduce discomfort, and remaining attentive to adverse effects. By regulating these parts of your treatment, you may ensure your drugs work correctly while making your digestive system as pleasant as possible.

Potential Side Effects of Medications

While treatments for stomach ulcers are frequently beneficial, they can also cause adverse effects. Recognizing these side effects and understanding how to manage them is critical to your comfort and safety. This section discusses frequent side effects such as allergic reactions, digestive difficulties from antibiotics, and the need to consult with your doctor if symptoms continue.

Recognizing Allergic Reactions.

While uncommon, allergic responses to ulcer medicines can be severe and necessitate emergency medical intervention. Antibiotics, PPIs, and H2 blockers can also cause allergies, so be mindful of the warning signals.

Common symptoms of an allergic reaction:

- Skin Rash or Hives are itchy, red, or swollen skin spots.

- Swelling of the cheeks, lips, tongue, or throat might cause trouble breathing.

- **Difficulty breathing or wheezing:** A dangerous symptom requiring immediate medical intervention.

- Dizziness or fainting is a severe response that should be reported promptly.

If you develop any of these symptoms, stop taking the drug and seek medical attention immediately. Before beginning therapy, advise your healthcare practitioner of any known allergies.

Managing Digestive Issues Caused By Antibiotics

Antibiotics for H. pylori might induce stomach problems such as nausea, diarrhea, and bloating. These adverse effects occur because antibiotics might upset the balance of beneficial microorganisms in the gut.

Tips to Manage Digestive Issues:

- *Stay Hydrated:* Drink plenty of fluids to avoid dehydration, particularly if you have diarrhea.

- *Take probiotics.* Probiotic supplements and probiotic-rich foods, such as yogurt and kefir, can help replace healthy bacteria in the stomach and alleviate antibiotic-related digestive difficulties.

- *Eat small, bland meals.* Choose readily digestible foods such as plain rice, bananas, or applesauce to ease an upset stomach.

- *Antibiotics with Probiotics:* Take probiotics a few hours after your antibiotic dose to enhance their effectiveness.

While specific digestive side effects are typical and tolerable, please notify your doctor if you experience severe or persistent symptoms.

It is critical to discuss with your doctor if your symptoms do not improve or if you have new or severe side effects. Persistent symptoms may suggest that your treatment strategy needs modification.

When To Contact Your Doctor:

- *Continued Pain or Discomfort:* If your ulcer symptoms persist despite treatment, your doctor may need to change your medications or consider other options.
- *Severe Side Effects:* Symptoms such as persistent diarrhea, vomiting, or severe abdominal discomfort should be reported immediately.
- *Worsening Symptoms:* If your condition deteriorates or new symptoms arise, seek medical attention.
- Regular follow-ups with your healthcare practitioner ensure your therapy is successful and well-tolerated.

Combining Medical Treatment and Alternative Therapies

Many people find relief for ulcer symptoms by combining medical and alternative remedies. Acupuncture, herbal medicine, and massage are complementary therapies that can help with general digestive health. However, you must consult your healthcare physician before beginning any alternative treatment.

Acupuncture and Massage for Ulcer Relief

Acupuncture and massage therapy are common alternative treatments that can help alleviate ulcer-related symptoms, including pain and tension.

Acupuncture is a traditional Chinese medicine procedure that involves inserting tiny needles into particular places on the body to stimulate energy flow and relieve pain. It may also help reduce stress, which can lead to ulcer symptoms, and increase overall calm.

Massage therapy can help relieve stress and muscle tension, which can contribute to stomach problems. Massage and other relaxation techniques can reduce stress hormone levels and improve digestion, indirectly aiding ulcer repair.

These therapies can be effective as part of a comprehensive ulcer care strategy, but they should be used in conjunction with, not instead of, medical treatments.

Herbal Medicine for Digestion.

Herbal remedies have long been used to improve digestion and calm the stomach lining. Certain herbs, such as chamomile, peppermint, and ginger, have anti-inflammatory effects that can help with indigestion and nausea.

- Chamomile tea, known for its relaxing properties, can help soothe and reduce inflammation in the digestive tract.
- **Peppermint:** While peppermint can help with bloating and gas, it should be used cautiously because it may relax the lower esophageal sphincter and aggravate acid reflux in certain people.
- **Ginger:** Ginger helps relieve nausea and improve healthy digestion, making it an excellent complement to an ulcer-friendly diet.

Always consult with your doctor before using herbal medicines since some herbs can interact with prescriptions or cause unwanted effects.

Consulting a Healthcare Provider about Alternative Treatments

Before beginning any alternative therapies, please consult your healthcare physician to confirm they are safe and will not conflict with your existing treatment plan.

Considerations for Consulting with Your Doctor:

Discuss potential interactions: Some natural treatments or supplements may interact with pharmaceuticals or worsen symptoms.

- *Develop a holistic treatment plan:* Work with your doctor to create a complete treatment plan that includes medical and alternative therapy to help your ulcer heal.

- *Monitor for effectiveness:* Track any changes in your symptoms and report them to your doctor to determine the efficacy of your treatment strategy.

Combining medical treatments with carefully selected alternative therapies can achieve a well-rounded approach to stomach ulcer management and long-term digestive health.

Breakfast Recipes

1. Banana Oatmeal

2. Soft-boiled eggs with Whole Wheat Toast

3. Avocado Toast on Whole Grain Bread

4. Yogurt and Honey Parfait

5. Smoothie with Almond Milk

6. Rice Porridge with Honey

7. Apple Cinnamon Overnight Oats

8. Mashed Sweet Potato Breakfast Bowl

9. Soft Banana Pancakes

10. Cottage Cheese with Soft Fruits

11. Warm Quinoa Breakfast Bowl with Almond Milk

12. Steamed Veggie Omelet

13. Chia Seed Pudding with Berries

14. Applesauce and Peanut Butter on Rice Cakes

15. Millet Porridge with Warm Spices (like cinnamon)

1. Banana Oatmeal

<u>INGREDIENTS</u>

- 1/2 cup rolled oats.
- One banana, sliced
- 1 tablespoon honey (optional for extra sweetness)
- 1 cup water or almond milk (or any milk you want)
- A pinch of cinnamon (optional to add flavor)

<u>INSTRUCTIONS:</u>

- In a medium saucepan, heat the water or almond milk until it boils.
- Add the rolled oats to the boiling liquid and lower to a simmer.
- Cook the oats for 5-7 minutes, stirring occasionally, until mushy and have absorbed most of the liquid.
- Remove the pot from the heat and allow the oatmeal to sit for a minute to thicken.
- Transfer the cooked oatmeal to a bowl.
- Top with sliced bananas and drizzle with honey for a delicious finish.
- Sprinkle a pinch of cinnamon over the top for extra flavor.
- Serve warm for a relaxing, ulcer-friendly breakfast.

Tips:

Use almond milk or another dairy-free alternative to add extra richness.

If you like a smoother texture, mash some banana slices into the oatmeal as it cooks.

2. *Soft-boiled eggs on whole wheat toast*

INGREDIENTS

- 2 eggs
- 1–2 slices of whole wheat bread
- A pinch of salt is optional.

INSTRUCTIONS

- Fill a small saucepan with water and heat to a low boil.
- To prevent cracking, gently add the eggs to the boiling water with a spoon.
- Boil the eggs for 5-6 minutes for a soft, runny yolk and 7-8 minutes for a little harder yolk.
- While the eggs boil, toast the whole wheat bread to the desired crispness.
- When the eggs are cooked, remove them from the boiling water and place them in cold water to halt the cooking process.
- Peel the eggs and serve beside the toasted whole wheat bread.
- Sprinkle a touch of salt over the eggs for extra taste.
- Enjoy a simple, protein-rich, and relaxing breakfast.

Tips:

If you have a sensitive stomach, avoid putting butter on toast.

To simplify digestion, lightly mash the eggs and put them on toast.

3. *Avocado Toast with Whole Grain Bread*

INGREDIENTS

- 1/2 ripe avocado.
- 1–2 slices of whole-grain bread
- A pinch of salt is optional.
- A sprinkle of olive oil is optional.

- Fresh herbs, such as chopped parsley or cilantro, are optional for extra taste.

INSTRUCTIONS:

- Toast the whole-grain bread to your desired level of crispness.
- While the bread is toasting, scoop out the avocado flesh and mash it in a bowl with a fork until smooth or somewhat chunky, as desired.
- Spread the mashed avocado equally on the toasted bread slices.
- To improve the flavor of the avocado, sprinkle it with salt.
- Drizzle a small quantity of olive oil over the toast and top with fresh herbs for added flavor.
- Serve immediately and enjoy this nutritious, ulcer-friendly breakfast.

Tips:

If you want a smoother avocado spread, mix it with olive oil.

Avoid spicy toppings or acidic components like lemon juice if you have a sensitive stomach.

4. Yogurt and honey parfait

INGREDIENTS

- 1 cup of plain yogurt (ideally low-fat or Greek yogurt for extra protein)
- 1 tablespoon honey Soft fruits, such as sliced bananas, blueberries, or strawberries.
- 1/4 cup granola or chopped nuts (optional, but only if tolerated)

INSTRUCTIONS

- In a glass or dish, spread a layer of plain yogurt.
- Drizzle a little honey over the yogurt to add natural sweetness.
- Add a layer of your preferred soft fruits, such as sliced bananas or blueberries.

- Repeat the layers until all the yogurt and fruit have been utilized, then sprinkle with honey on top.
- Add a bit of granola or chopped nuts for texture if preferred and tolerated.
- Serve immediately and relish this refreshing, ulcer-friendly parfait.

Tips:

Choose soft, nonacidic fruits such as bananas or cooked apples to avoid stomach distress.

If granola or nuts upset your stomach, skip them and stick with the soft fruit and yogurt combination.

If you are allergic to dairy, go for a dairy-free yogurt substitute.

5. Smoothie with Almond Milk

<u>INGREDIENTS</u>

- 1 banana.
- 1/2 cup spinach, fresh or frozen.
- 1/2 cup blueberries, fresh or frozen.
- 1 cup unsweetened almond milk (or your preferred milk option)
- 1 tablespoon honey (optional for extra sweetness)

<u>INSTRUCTIONS</u>

- Place the banana, spinach, blueberries, and almond milk in a blender.
- Blend until smooth and creamy. If the smoothie is too thick, add almond milk and combine until it reaches the required consistency.
- Taste the smoothie; if you want it sweeter, add honey and blend again.
- Pour the smoothie into a glass and serve it immediately.

Tips:

Ripe bananas provide natural sweetness and make the smoothie simpler to stomach.

Frozen blueberries can make the smoothie even more pleasant, but fresh berries are ideal for a room-temperature drink.

If you wish to add protein, use a modest amount of protein powder that is easy on your stomach.

6. Rice Porridge with Honey

INGREDIENTS

- 1/2 cup white rice.
- 4 cups water
- 1 tablespoon honey (or to taste).
- A pinch of salt (optional).
- Soft fruits, such as sliced bananas or boiled apples, are optional for added nourishment.

INSTRUCTIONS

- To remove extra starch, rinse the rice in cold water until it clears.
- In a medium saucepan, combine rice and water. Bring to the boil over medium heat.
- Once boiling, reduce the heat to low and simmer, stirring occasionally, until the rice is mushy and porridge-like. This will take approximately 45 to 60 minutes.
- If preferred, add a pinch of salt and thoroughly stir.
- Remove the porridge from the heat once it has reached your desired consistency.
- Serve heated in a bowl and drizzle with honey for a natural sweetener.
- Top with soft fruits, such as sliced bananas or baked apples, for extra flavor and nutrition.

Tips:

Use white rice instead of brown rice because it is easier to digest and less harsh on the stomach.

Adjust the amount of water until the porridge reaches the desired consistency. Near the conclusion of cooking, add a little additional water or milk (dairy-free options are available).

7. Apple Cinnamon Overnight Oats

<u>INGREDIENTS</u>

- 1/2 cup rolled oats.
- 1/2 cup of unsweetened almond milk (or your chosen milk).
- 1/4 cup unsweetened applesauce.
- 1/4 teaspoon of ground cinnamon.
- 1 tablespoon honey or maple syrup (optional for extra sweetness)
- 1/4 cup sliced soft apples (optional for topping).

<u>INSTRUCTIONS:</u>

- Mix the rolled oats, almond milk, applesauce, and ground cinnamon in a mason jar or dish.
- Stir thoroughly to ensure all oats are fully coated and combined with the liquid.
- To sweeten your oats, add honey or maple syrup and mix again.
- Cover the jar or dish and chill overnight, or at least 4 hours, to let the oats soften and absorb the flavors.
- In the morning, mix the oats thoroughly. If the consistency is too thick, add more milk to thin it.
- If desired, top with chopped soft apples to add texture and flavor.
- Enjoy this tasty, ulcer-friendly breakfast from the fridge or slightly reheated.

Tips:

To make the recipe easier on your stomach, use unsweetened applesauce and adjust the sweetness to your liking.

If you like warm oatmeal, heat it briefly in the microwave or stove before adding the apple topping.

8. Mashed Sweet Potato Breakfast Bowl

INGREDIENTS

- 1 medium sweet potato (about 1 cup mashed).
- 1/4 cup of unsweetened almond milk (or your chosen milk).
- 1 tablespoon nut butter (almond, peanut, or cashew)
- 1 tablespoon of maple syrup or honey (optional for sweetness)
- 1/2 teaspoon ground cinnamon (to taste)

Toppings (choose your favorite):

- Sliced bananas
- Chopped nuts (such as walnuts and pecans)
- Dried fruit (such as raisins and cranberries)
- Chia seed or flaxseed
- Greek yogurt (for more protein).

INSTRUCTIONS

- Peel and dice the sweet potato. Cook or steam until tender, about 15-20 minutes. Alternatively, microwave until soft.
- Drain the sweet potato (if boiled) and place it in a mixing bowl. Combine the almond milk, nut butter, maple syrup or honey (if using), and ground cinnamon. Mash until smooth and creamy, adjusting the milk to the appropriate consistency.

- Transfer the mashed sweet potato mixture to a bowl.
- Optional toppings include sliced bananas, chopped almonds, dried fruit, seeds, and a dollop of Greek yogurt.
- Enjoy warm for a soothing and nutritious breakfast!

Tips:

Make mashed sweet potatoes and refrigerate for a quick breakfast throughout the week.

For more taste, try using various spices like nutmeg or ginger.

To improve the protein content, add a scoop of protein powder or Greek yogurt to the mashed sweet potato mixture.

9. Soft Banana Pancakes

INGREDIENTS

- 1/2 cup of rolled oats.
- 1/2 cup of unsweetened almond milk (or your chosen milk).
- 1/4 cup unsweetened applesauce.
- 1/4 teaspoon of ground cinnamon.
- 1 tablespoon honey or maple syrup (optional for extra sweetness)
- 1/4 cup sliced soft apples (optional for topping).

INSTRUCTIONS

- Mix the rolled oats, almond milk, applesauce, and ground cinnamon in a mason jar or dish.
- Stir thoroughly to ensure all oats are fully coated and combined with the liquid.
- To sweeten your oats, add honey or maple syrup and mix again.

- Cover the jar or dish and chill overnight, or at least 4 hours, to let the oats to soften and absorb the flavors.

- In the morning, mix the oats thoroughly. If the consistency is too thick, add more milk to thin it.

- If desired, top with chopped soft apples to add texture and flavor.

- Enjoy this tasty, ulcer-friendly breakfast from the fridge or slightly reheated.

Tips:

To make the recipe easier on your stomach, use unsweetened applesauce and adjust the sweetness to your liking.

If you like warm oatmeal, heat it briefly in the microwave or stove before adding the apple topping.

10. Cottage Cheese with Soft Fruits

INGREDIENTS

- 1 cup cottage cheese, either low-fat or full-fat.

- One ripe banana cut

- 1/2 cup chopped ripe peaches, either fresh or canned.

- 1/2 cup berries (blueberries, raspberries, or strawberries).

- 1 tablespoon honey or maple syrup (optional for extra sweetness)

- 1/4 teaspoon ground cinnamon (optional for flavoring)

- **Optional topping:** chopped nuts or seeds (e.g., walnuts, almonds, chia seeds).

INSTRUCTIONS

- In a bowl, combine the cottage cheese.

- Top the cottage cheese with banana slices, diced peaches, and berries.

- Drizzle honey or maple syrup over the fruits for extra richness. Sprinkle with ground cinnamon for added taste.

- Top with chopped nuts or seeds for extra texture and nutrition if desired.

- Consume immediately as a refreshing breakfast or snack.

Tips:

Experiment with additional soft fruits such as mango, kiwi, or plums to suit your taste and season.

This recipe is high in protein from cottage cheese, making it an excellent choice for a filling supper.

Prepare individual servings in jars for a simple grab-and-go breakfast or snack all week.

11. Warm Quinoa Breakfast Bowl with Almond Milk

<u>INGREDIENTS</u>

- 1 cup cooked quinoa (equivalent to 1/3 cup dry quinoa cooked).
- 1 cup of unsweetened almond milk (or your chosen milk).
- 1 tablespoon maple syrup or honey (optional for extra sweetness)
- 1/2 teaspoon of vanilla extract (optional)
- 1/2 teaspoon ground cinnamon (to taste)
- 1/2 cup of chopped soft fruits (bananas, peaches, or berries)
- Top with chopped nuts or seeds (almonds, walnuts, or chia seeds).
- Optional toppings include shredded coconut, nut butter, and yogurt.

<u>INSTRUCTIONS</u>

- Combine the cooked quinoa and almond milk in a saucepan over medium heat. Stir thoroughly and bring to a medium simmer.
- Mix in the maple syrup or honey (if using), vanilla essence, and ground cinnamon. Stir to mix, then simmer for 3-5 minutes until well cooked and creamy.
- Remove from the fire and place the warm quinoa mixture in a bowl.

- Garnish with diced soft fruits and chopped nuts or seeds. Add whatever other toppings you choose.
- Serve warm and savor your nutritious breakfast bowl!

Tips:

Cooked quinoa: Prepare quinoa ahead of time and refrigerate it for easy assembly in the morning.

Flavor Variations: Try adding spices such as nutmeg and cardamom for added diversity.

Meal Prep: Make a batch of quinoa and dish it out for multiple breakfasts during the week.

12. Steamed Veggie Omelet

<u>INGREDIENTS</u>

- Two big eggs.
- 1/4 cup milk (or your favorite milk)
- 1/4 cup sliced bell peppers, any color
- 1/4 cup chopped spinach, fresh or frozen.
- 1/4 cup chopped tomatoes.
- 1/4 cup chopped onions.
- Add salt and pepper to taste.
- one tablespoon olive oil (to grease)
- Optional toppings include shredded cheese, herbs (such as chives or parsley), and avocado slices.

INSTRUCTIONS

- In a mixing dish, combine diced bell peppers, spinach, tomatoes, and onions. Set aside.

- Mix the eggs, milk, salt, and pepper in a separate bowl until well blended.

- Gently incorporate the prepared vegetables into the egg mixture.

- Lightly coat a heatproof dish or small pan with olive oil. Pour the egg and vegetable mixture into the dish.

- Fill a pot with water and heat to a simmer. Place a steaming rack or oven-safe dish over the pot, ensuring it does not touch the water.

- Cover the pot and steam the omelet for 10-15 minutes, or until the eggs are firm.

- Carefully remove the dish from the pot and let it cool for a minute before slicing and serving. Optional toppings include shredded cheese, fresh herbs, and avocado slices.

Tips:

Use any vegetables on hand, including zucchini, mushrooms, and broccoli.

You can make the vegetable mixture the night before to save time in the morning.

Use spices such as garlic powder, paprika, or red pepper flakes for added taste.

13. Chia Seed Pudding with Berries

INGREDIENTS

- 1/4 cup of chia seeds.

- 1 cup of unsweetened almond milk (or your chosen milk).

- 1 tablespoon of maple syrup or honey (optional for sweetness)

- 1/2 teaspoon of vanilla extract (optional)

- 1/2 cup mixed berries (strawberries, blueberries, raspberries, or blackberries).

- Toppings (Optional) sliced banana, nuts or granola.

<u>**INSTRUCTIONS**</u>

- In a mixing bowl, blend chia seeds, almond milk, maple syrup or honey (if using), and vanilla essence. Stir well to avoid clumps.

- Cover the bowl and chill for at least 2 hours, preferably overnight, to allow the chia seeds to absorb the liquid and thicken into a pudding-like texture.

- Once the pudding has set, give it a good stir. If it's too thick, add more almond milk to achieve the correct consistency.

- Serve the chia pudding in bowls or jars, topped with mixed berries and any additional toppings you choose.

Tips:

Make Ahead: Chia seed pudding can be made ahead of time and refrigerated for up to 5 days, making it ideal for a quick breakfast or snack.

Flavor variations: Experiment with different flavors by adding cocoa powder, cinnamon, or extracts such as almond or coconut.

Sweetness Adjustment: Use more or less maple syrup or honey to achieve the desired sweetness.

14. Applesauce and Peanut Butter on Rice Cakes

<u>**INGREDIENTS**</u>

- Rice cakes (simple or seasoned to taste).
- 1/2 cup unsweetened applesauce.
- 2 tablespoons peanut butter (or your favorite nut butter)
- Cinnamon (optional to sprinkle)
- Chopped nuts or seeds (optional for topping)
- Sliced bananas or other fruits (optional for extra flavor)

- **Prepare the rice cakes:** Place the rice cakes flat on a platter or cutting board.
- **Spread Peanut Butter:** Evenly distribute 1 tablespoon peanut butter onto each rice cake.
- Top the peanut butter with a big scoop of unsweetened applesauce.
- **Toppings:** For added taste and texture, sprinkle with cinnamon and top with chopped nuts, seeds, or sliced fruits.
- Serve immediately as a nutritious snack or quick breakfast.

Tips:

Alternatives to peanut butter include almond butter, cashew butter, and sunflower seed butter, which have various flavor profiles.

Rice Cake Options: Choose rice cakes made with brown rice, whole grain, or flavored variants.

Meal Prep: Make multiple rice cakes ahead of time and keep in an airtight container for a quick snack during the week.

15. Millet Porridge with Warm Spices (like cinnamon)

INGREDIENTS

- 1 cup washed millet.
- 3 cups of water (or almond milk for creamier porridge).
- 1/2 teaspoon ground cinnamon (or more as desired)
- 1/4 teaspoon of ground nutmeg (optional)
- 1 tablespoon of maple syrup or honey (optional for sweetness)
- 1/2 cup of diced soft fruits (bananas, apples, or pears)
- Top with chopped nuts or seeds (such as walnuts, almonds, or pumpkin seeds).
- A pinch of salt.

<u>**INSTRUCTIONS**</u>

- Combine the washed millet with water (or almond milk) and a pinch of salt in a medium saucepan. Bring to a boil over medium high heat.
- Once boiling, decrease the heat to low, cover, and allow it simmer for 15-20 minutes, or until the millet is soft and the liquid has been absorbed.
- Add the ground cinnamon, nutmeg (if using), and maple syrup or honey (as desired). Mix thoroughly to mix.
- Spoon the porridge into bowls. For extra texture and nutrients, top with diced soft fruits and chopped nuts or seeds.
- Serve warm and savor your nutritious breakfast!

Tip:

Rinse millet before cooking to remove bitterness and increase flavor.

To make a creamier porridge, increase the liquid or add a drop of milk while cooking.

Experiment with other spices, such as ginger or cardamom, to create diverse flavor profiles.

<u>**Lunch Recipes**</u>

1. Grilled Chicken and Vegetable Wrap

2. Baked Salmon with Steamed Broccoli and Quinoa

3. Turkey and Avocado Sandwich on Whole Wheat Bread

4. Vegetable and Lentil Soup

5. Rice and Black Bean Bowl with Fresh Herbs

6. Sautéed Zucchini and Spinach with Brown Rice

7. Simple Chicken and Sweet Potato Bake

8. Quinoa Salad with Cucumber, Tomato, and Olive Oil

9. Tofu Stir-Fry with Soft Vegetables and Rice Noodles

10. Baked Cod with Mashed Cauliflower and Green Beans

1. Grilled Chicken and Vegetable Wrap

<u>INGREDIENTS</u>

* 1 boneless and skinless chicken breast.

* 1 whole wheat wrap or spinach tortilla

* 1/2 cup baby spinach or shredded lettuce.

* 1/4 cup shredded carrots.

* 1/4 cup diced cucumber.

* 1/4 avocado, sliced

* Olive Oil for Grilling

* Salt and pepper (optional; to taste)

* A small spray of olive oil or a mild yogurt-based dressing is optional.

<u>INSTRUCTIONS</u>

* If desired, season the chicken breasts lightly with salt and pepper.

* Brush a tiny quantity of olive oil into a grill pan or skillet set over medium heat.

* Grill the chicken breasts on each side for 6-7 minutes, or until thoroughly cooked and no longer pink in the center. Internal temperature should be 165°F (74°C).

* Remove the chicken from the pan and let aside for a few minutes before slicing into thin strips.

* Place the whole wheat or spinach wrap on a flat surface.

* Add shredded lettuce or baby spinach, carrots, diced cucumber, and sliced avocado to the wrap.

* Place the grilled chicken strips on top of the veggies.

* If preferred, drizzle the filling with olive oil or a mild yogurt dressing.

* Fold in the sides of the wrap and roll it securely.

* Cut in half and serve immediately for a healthy, ulcer-friendly lunch.

Tips:

Avoid spicy sauces and strong flavors to make the wrap easier on the stomach.

You can tailor the vegetables to your taste or tolerance, opting for soft, readily digested alternatives.

2. Baked Salmon with Steamed Broccoli and Quinoa

INGREDIENTS

- 1 salmon fillet (about 4-6 ounces)
- 1 cup of broccoli florets.
- 1/2 cup quinoa.
- 1 tablespoon of olive oil.
- Salt and pepper (optional; to taste)
- Fresh lemon slices (optional for garnish).

INSTRUCTIONS

- Rinse the quinoa with cool water to remove any bitterness.
- Add the quinoa, 1 cup of water, and a teaspoon of salt to taste in a medium saucepan.
- Bring to a boil, then reduce heat, cover, and simmer for 15 minutes, or until the quinoa is fluffy and the water has been absorbed. Set aside.
- Preheat the oven to 375°F (190° C).
- Place the salmon fillet on a baking pan covered with parchment paper.
- Drizzle olive oil over the fish and season with salt and pepper as desired.
- Bake for 12-15 minutes until the salmon flaked easily with a fork.
- While baking the salmon, boil a pot of water and set a steamer basket over it.
- Place the broccoli florets in the steamer basket, cover, and steam for 5-7 minutes until tender yet brilliant green.
- Serve the baked salmon with steamed broccoli and a scoop of cooked quinoa.

- If preferred, garnish with fresh lemon slices, or drizzle with olive oil to enhance the flavor of the broccoli and quinoa.

Tips:

Avoid flavoring the salmon with spicy or acidic sauces to keep the meal stomach-friendly.

If your stomach can handle citrus, pour some lemon juice over the salmon for a refreshing, mild flavor.

3. Turkey and Avocado Sandwich on Whole Wheat Bread

INGREDIENTS

- two slices of whole-wheat bread
- 4-6 slices of cooked turkey breast (low-sodium, deli-style, roasted)
- 1/2 avocado (sliced or mashed)
- 1-2 slices of tomato (optional, but well accepted)
- A handful of spinach or lettuce.
- A drizzle of olive oil or a little spread of mild mustard is optional.
- Salt and pepper (optional; to taste)

INSTRUCTIONS

- To add a little crunch, lightly toast the whole wheat bread.
- Spread the mashed or sliced avocado evenly on one slice of bread.
- Layer turkey slices on top of the avocado.
- Place the lettuce, spinach, and tomato slices (if used) on the turkey.
- Drizzle with olive oil or a little smear of mustard for added flavor—season with salt and pepper to taste.
- Top with the second slice of bread, cut the sandwich in two and serve.

Tips:

To avoid discomfort caused by high salt, use low-sodium turkey breast.

Avoid spicy sauces and acidic spreads that might irritate the stomach.

Add other vegetables like sliced cucumber or shredded carrots for extra crunch and nutrients.

4. Vegetable and Lentil Soup

INGREDIENTS

- 1 cup red or green lentils, rinsed
- 1 carrot, diced
- 1 zucchini, diced
- 1 celery stalk, diced
- 1 small potato, peeled and diced
- 1/2 onion, finely chopped
- 3 cloves garlic, minced
- 6 cups low-sodium vegetable broth or water
- 1 tablespoon olive oil
- 1 teaspoon dried thyme or oregano (optional)
- Salt and pepper (optional, to taste)

INSTRUCTIONS

- Heat the olive oil in a big pot over medium heat. Add the chopped onion and garlic, and sauté until the onion becomes translucent, about 3-5 minutes.
- Add the chopped carrot, celery, potato, and zucchini to the pot. Sauté for another 5 minutes to soften the veggies slightly.
- Add the rinsed lentils to the pot and stir well to mix.

- Pour the veggie broth or water and add the dried thyme or oregano. Stir well and bring to a boil.

- Reduce the heat to low, cover, and simmer for 25-30 minutes or until the lentils and veggies are tender.

- Season with salt and pepper to taste, if preferred. Adjust the thickness of the soup by adding more broth or water if needed.

- Serve warm with a slice of whole wheat bread or a side of soft crackers for a filling, ulcer-friendly lunch.

Tips:

Avoid using solid seasonings to keep the soup gentle on your stomach.

You can blend part of the soup for a creamier texture but leave some chunks for added structure.

5. Rice and Black Bean Bowl with Fresh Herbs

INGREDIENTS

- 1 cup red or green lentils, rinsed 1 carrot, diced 1 zucchini, diced 1 celery stalk, diced 1 small potato, peeled and diced 1/2 onion, finely chopped 3 cloves garlic, minced

- 6 cups low-sodium veggie broth or water

- 1 tablespoon olive oil

- 1 teaspoon dried thyme or oregano (optional)

- Salt and pepper (extra, to taste)

- 1 cup cooked brown or white rice

- 1 can of black beans, drained and washed

- 1/2 cup chopped cucumber

- 1/2 cup diced bell pepper (use yellow or red for a milder taste)

- 1/4 cup chopped fresh herbs (such as cilantro or parsley)

- 1 tablespoon olive oil

- Salt and pepper (extra, to taste)

- Fresh lime wedges (optional, if well handled)

INSTRUCTIONS

- In a big mixing bowl, combine the cooked rice and black beans.

- Add the diced cucumber and bell pepper, mixing gently to combine.

- Drizzle the olive oil over the mixture and stir well to coat everything evenly.

- Add the chopped fresh herbs and gently mix again.

- Season with salt and pepper to taste, if preferred.

- Serve the rice and black bean bowl warm or at room temperature. Optionally, add a squeeze of fresh lime juice for a light, zesty flavor if your stomach can handle citrus.

Tips:

To make this dish even more soothing, try using white rice instead of brown rice, as it's easier to digest.

Avoid adding spicy sauces or seasonings to make the dish ulcer-friendly.

You can customize the bowl by adding other soft veggies, such as diced avocado, for added creaminess.

6. Sautéed Zucchini and Spinach with Brown Rice

INGREDIENTS

- 1 cup cooked brown rice

- 1 medium zucchini, chopped into half-moons

- 2 cups fresh spinach leaves

- 2 tablespoons olive oil

- 2 cloves garlic, minced

- Salt and pepper (extra, to taste)

- Fresh lemon wedges (optional, if well handled)

INSTRUCTIONS

- Heat the olive oil in a big skillet over medium heat.

- Add the minced garlic and sauté for 1-2 minutes until fragrant, being careful not to burn it.

- Add the sliced zucchini to the pan and cook for 5-7 minutes, stirring occasionally, until the zucchini is tender and lightly golden.

- Add the fresh spinach to the pan and cook for another 2-3 minutes, or until the spinach wilts.

- Season with salt and pepper to taste, if preferred.

- Serve the sautéed zucchini and spinach over warm, cooked brown rice bed.

- Optionally, add fresh lemon juice for a light, refreshing flavor if your stomach can handle citrus.

Tips:

You can use garlic powder instead of fresh garlic if you prefer a milder garlic taste.

White rice can be used instead of brown rice for better digestion.

For extra nutrients and variety, feel free to add other soft veggies, such as diced bell pepper.

7. Simple Chicken and Sweet Potato Bake

INGREDIENTS

- 2 boneless and skinless chicken breasts.

- 2 medium sweet potatoes, peeled and sliced into 1 inch cubes.

- 1 tablespoon of olive oil.

- 1 teaspoon dried thyme or rosemary (optional).
- Salt and pepper (optional; to taste)

INSTRUCTIONS

- Preheat the oven to 375°F (190° C).
- Put the cubed sweet potatoes in a baking dish and drizzle with half of the olive oil. Season with dried thyme or rosemary, as well as a touch of salt and pepper to taste. Toss to coat evenly.
- Put the chicken breasts on top of the sweet potatoes in the baking dish. Drizzle the remaining olive oil over the chicken, then season with salt and pepper as needed.
- Cover the baking dish with aluminum foil to keep the contents moist, and bake for 25-30 minutes.
- Remove the foil and bake for another 10-15 minutes, or until the chicken is thoroughly cooked (internal temperature of 165°F or 74°C) and the sweet potatoes are soft.
- Allow the dish to cool for a few minutes before serving.

Tips:

For added variation, add other soft veggies to the baking dish, such as sliced carrots or zucchini.

To make the food easier on the stomach, avoid using hot flavors or acidic ingredients.

This meal can be prepared ahead of time and refrigerated for simple reheating.

8. *Quinoa Salad with Cucumber, Tomato, and Olive Oil*

INGREDIENTS

- 1 cup cooked quinoa
- 1/2 cup diced cucumber
- 1/2 cup diced tomatoes (seeds removed if preferred for easier digestion)
- 1/4 cup chopped fresh parsley or cilantro
- 2 tablespoons olive oil
- Salt and pepper (optional, to taste)
- Fresh lemon juice (optional, if well tolerated)

INSTRUCTIONS

- In a large mixing bowl, combine the cooked quinoa, diced cucumber, diced tomatoes, and chopped fresh parsley or cilantro.
- Drizzle the olive oil over the salad and toss well to coat all the ingredients evenly.
- Season with salt and pepper to taste, if desired.
- If your stomach can tolerate it, add a splash of fresh lemon juice for extra flavor.
- Serve the quinoa salad chilled or at room temperature for a refreshing, ulcer-friendly lunch.

Tips:

To make the salad even more soothing, you can peel the cucumber and remove the seeds from the tomatoes.

Avoid adding strong or spicy seasonings to keep the dish gentle on the stomach.

This salad can be stored in the refrigerator for up to 2 days, making it a convenient option for meal prep.

9. Tofu Stir-Fry with Soft Vegetables and Rice Noodles

INGREDIENTS

- 1 brick of firm tofu, drained and cubed.
- 1 cup sliced soft vegetables, such as bell peppers, zucchini, carrots, or bok choy.
- 2 cups cooked rice noodles.
- 2 tablespoons olive or sesame oil.
- 2 garlic cloves, minced
- 2 tablespoons of low-sodium soy sauce or tamari.
- 1 tablespoon honey or maple syrup (optional sweetener)
- Salt and pepper (optional; to taste)

INSTRUCTIONS

- Heat 1 tablespoon oil in a large skillet or wok over medium heat. Add the tofu cubes and cook for 5-7 minutes, rotating regularly, until golden brown all over. Remove the tofu from the skillet and set it aside.
- Add the last tablespoon of oil to the skillet. Sauté the minced garlic for 1-2 minutes, until fragrant.
- Add the sliced vegetables to the skillet and cook for 5-6 minutes, or until tender but still crunchy. You can add a splash of water if necessary to steam and soften the vegetables.
- Return the tofu to the skillet, then add the cooked rice noodles.
- Drizzle the stir-fry with low-sodium soy sauce or tamari, as well as the honey (if using). Toss everything well to mix, then heat through.
- Season with salt and pepper to taste.
- Serve the tofu stir-fry warm for a nutritious, ulcer-friendly supper.

Tips:

Use soft, easy-to-digest vegetables to make the meal pleasant on the stomach.

To avoid irritation, do not add hot sauces or chile oil.

If acceptable, sprinkle with sesame seeds or chopped green onions for added taste.

10. Baked Cod with Mashed Cauliflower and Green Beans

INGREDIENTS

- Two fillets of cod
- cauliflower, chopped into florets, one head of cauliflower
- olive oil, one tablespoon (plus additional olive oil for drizzling)
- a half cup of low-fat or unsweetened almond milk or milk
- 2 cups green beans, trimmed
- Salt and pepper (optional, to taste)
- Lemon wedges made from fresh lemons (optional, if well tolerated)

INSTRUCTIONS

- Bring a big saucepan of water to a boil and add the cauliflower florets.
- Cook for about 10-12 minutes, or until the cauliflower is soft and tender.
- Drain and transfer the cooked cauliflower to a blender or food processor.
- Add the olive oil and milk, and blend until smooth and creamy. Season with salt and pepper if required. Set aside.
- Preheat your oven to 375°F (190°C).
- Place the fish fillets on a baking pan lined with parchment paper. Drizzle with olive oil and season moderately with salt and pepper if preferred.
- Bake for 12-15 minutes, or until the fish is opaque and flakes readily with a fork.
- While the cod is baking, cook the green beans in a steamer basket over boiling water for about 5-7 minutes, or until soft but still brilliant green.

- Season with a bit of salt and a dab of olive oil, if desired.
- Serve the baked cod atop a big scoop of mashed cauliflower and steaming green beans.
- Optionally, sprinkle a squeeze of fresh lemon juice over the fish for a bit of brightness, if your stomach can accept citrus.

Tips:

You can substitute cod with another mild white fish like tilapia or haddock if preferred.

For extra taste, scatter fresh herbs such as parsley or dill over the fish before serving.

The mashed cauliflower can be made creamier by adding a bit extra milk or olive oil if needed.

<u>**Dinner Recipes**</u>

1. Herb-Baked Chicken Breast with Roasted Sweet Potatoes and Steamed Asparagus
2. Mild Vegetable Curry with Coconut Milk and Brown Rice
3. Turkey Meatballs in a Light Tomato Sauce with Whole Wheat Pasta
4. Baked Tilapia with Soft Carrot and Zucchini Medley
5. Stuffed Bell Peppers with Quinoa, Spinach, and Feta Cheese
6. Simple Beef and Vegetable Stew with Soft Potatoes and Carrots
7. Grilled Shrimp with Mashed Butternut Squash and Green Peas
8. Vegetable Risotto with Mushrooms, Spinach, and Parmesan Cheese
9. Lentil and Vegetable Shepherd's Pie with Mashed Potato Topping
10. Baked Eggplant Parmesan (Lightly Breaded) with a Side Salad

1. *Herb-Baked Chicken Breast with Roasted Sweet Potatoes and Steamed Asparagus*

INGREDIENTS

- 2 boneless, skinless chicken breasts
- 2 medium sweet potatoes, peeled and cubed 1 bunch of asparagus, trimmed 3 tablespoons olive oil, divided 1 teaspoon dried herbs (such as thyme, rosemary, or oregano)
- Salt and pepper (optional, to taste)

INSTRUCTIONS

- Preheat your oven to 375°F (190°C).
- Place the chicken breasts on a baking pan lined with parchment paper.
- Drizzle 1 tablespoon of olive oil over the chicken and season with dried herbs, salt, and pepper if preferred.
- Rub the herbs and oil evenly over the chicken breasts.
- Set aside while you prepare the sweet potatoes.
- Place the diced sweet potatoes on another baking sheet or in a baking dish.
- Drizzle 1 tablespoon of olive oil over the sweet potatoes and season with a bit of salt and pepper if preferred.
- Toss to coat the sweet potatoes evenly.
- Place the sweet potatoes in the oven and roast for 25-30 minutes, or until they are soft and slightly caramelized, tossing halfway through.
- Add the chicken breasts to the oven beside the sweet potatoes.
- Bake for 20-25 minutes, or until the chicken is cooked through and reaches an internal temperature of 165°F (74°C). The chicken should be juicy and tender.
- While the chicken and sweet potatoes are baking, bring a pot of water to a boil and lay a steamer basket over it.

- Add the asparagus to the steamer basket, cover, and steam for 5-7 minutes, or until the asparagus is tender but still brilliant green.
- Drizzle the steamed asparagus with the remaining 1 tablespoon of olive oil and season generously with salt if preferred.
- Serve the herb-baked chicken breasts with a side of roasted sweet potatoes and steamed asparagus for a balanced, ulcer-friendly dinner.

Tips:

If you like, you can marinate the chicken for 30 minutes in olive oil, herbs, and a little lemon juice (if your stomach tolerates citrus) for added flavor.

Avoid using strong spices or acidic sauces to keep the dish mild on your tummy.

2. Mild Vegetable Curry with Coconut Milk and Brown Rice

INGREDIENTS

- 1 tablespoon of olive or coconut oil.
- To prepare, finely slice 1 small onion, mince 2 garlic cloves, grate 1 inch of fresh ginger, dice 1 large carrot, dice 1 zucchini, and dice 1 bell pepper (yellow or red).
- 1 cup of cauliflower florets.
- 1 can (14 ounces) Light coconut milk.
- 1 cup low-sodium vegetable broth.
- 1 teaspoon of mild curry powder.
- 1/2 teaspoon turmeric.
- Salt and pepper (optional; to taste)
- Freshly chopped cilantro (optional for garnish)
- 2 cups of cooked brown rice.

INSTRUCTIONS:

- Prepare the brown rice according to the package directions. Set aside.

- In a big pan or saucepan, warm the olive or coconut oil over medium heat.
- Add the chopped onion and cook for 3-5 minutes, or until transparent.
- Add the minced garlic and grated ginger and simmer for another 1-2 minutes, or until fragrant.
- Place the diced carrot, zucchini, bell pepper, and cauliflower florets in the pot.
- Cook the vegetables for 5-7 minutes, stirring regularly, until they begin to soften.
- Add the coconut milk and spices.
- Add the light coconut milk and vegetable broth, stirring to mix.
- Add the mild curry powder and turmeric, and stir thoroughly.
- Season with a bit of salt and pepper as required.
- Simmer the curry.
- Cook the curry at a gentle simmer for 15-20 minutes, or until the veggies are soft.
- Taste and adjust seasoning as needed.
- Serve the mild vegetable curry on a bed of heated brown rice.
- If desired, garnish with freshly cut cilantro.

Tips:

Use a mild curry powder to keep the spice level moderate and easy on the stomach. Avoid spicy chili powders and hot sauces.

For further diversity, try adding additional soft vegetables like as spinach or green beans.

If you prefer a thicker curry, simmer for longer to reduce the liquid, or thicken with a slurry of cornstarch and water.

3. Turkey Meatballs in a Light Tomato Sauce with Whole Wheat Pasta

INGREDIENT

For the turkey meatballs:

- 1 pound ground turkey

- 1/2 cup whole wheat breadcrumbs.

- Ingredients: 1 egg and 2 minced garlic cloves.

- 1/4 cup finely chopped parsley.

- Salt and pepper (optional; to taste)

For the light tomato sauce:

- 1 tablespoon of olive oil.

- 1 small, finely chopped onion

- 2 garlic cloves, minced

- 1 can (14 ounces) Diced tomatoes (low sodium)

- 1/2 cup low-sodium chicken broth.

- One teaspoon dried basil or oregano.

- Salt and pepper (optional; to taste)

For serving:

- 8 ounces whole wheat pasta

- Fresh basil or parsley (optional for garnish).

- grated Parmesan cheese (optional)

INSTRUCTIONS

- Preheat the oven to 400 °F (200 °C).

- In a large mixing bowl, combine ground turkey, whole wheat breadcrumbs, egg, garlic, parsley, salt, and pepper.

- Mix thoroughly until all components are incorporated. Form small meatballs (approximately an inch in diameter) and lay them on a baking sheet coated with parchment paper.

- Bake the meatballs for 15-20 minutes, or until they are golden brown and fully cooked.

- While the meatballs bake, prepare the whole wheat spaghetti according to package directions. Drain and set aside.

- Heat the olive oil in a large skillet over medium heat. Add the chopped onion and cook for 3-5 minutes, or until transparent.

- Add the minced garlic and simmer for another 1-2 minutes, or until fragrant.

- Combine the diced tomatoes, chicken stock, and dried basil or oregano. Season with salt and pepper as desired.

- Simmer the sauce for 10-15 minutes, until it has reduced and thickened somewhat.

- Once the meatballs have finished baking, add them to the skillet with the tomato sauce.

- Gently toss to coat the meatballs with the sauce. Allow to boil in the sauce for 5-10 minutes to absorb the flavors.

- Serve the turkey meatballs with tomato sauce on a bed of whole wheat spaghetti.

- Garnish with fresh basil or parsley, then serve with grated Parmesan cheese.

Tips:

For a lighter sauce, use diced tomatoes with no salt or seasonings.

To make the dish easier on the stomach, avoid using hot flavors in the meatballs or sauce.

If whole wheat pasta is too heavy, use rice pasta or cooked quinoa instead.

4. Baked Tilapia with Soft Carrot and Zucchini Medley

<u>INGREDIENTS</u>

- Two tilapia fillets.
- Two medium carrots, peeled and cut into thin rounds.
- 1 medium zucchini, sliced into half moons.
- 2 tablespoons olive oil, divided.
- 1 teaspoon dry herbs (such thyme or oregano)
- Salt and pepper (optional; to taste)
- Fresh lemon wedges (optional if well tolerated).

<u>INSTRUCTIONS</u>

- Preheat the oven to 375°F (190° C).
- Put the tilapia fillets on a baking pan lined with parchment paper.
- Drizzle 1 tablespoon olive oil over the fillets, then season with dry herbs, salt, and pepper to taste.
- Set aside while you prepare the vegetables.
- In a large mixing basin, combine the sliced carrots and zucchini.
- Drizzle the remaining tablespoon olive oil over the vegetables and toss to coat evenly.
- Season with a bit of salt and pepper as required.
- Put the fish and vegetables in the oven. Bake for 15-20 minutes, or until the tilapia is thoroughly cooked and readily flaked with a fork, and the vegetables are soft.
- Serve the cooked tilapia with the soft carrot and zucchini medley as a side.
- If your stomach can handle citrus, pour some fresh lemon juice over the fish for a mild, zesty flavor.

Tips:

Tilapia is a mild, readily digestible fish, making it a good choice for persons with delicate digestive systems.

Before serving, sprinkle the fish with fresh parsley or dill to add flavor.

For more variation, add other soft vegetables to the mix, such as bell peppers or spinach.

5. Stuffed Bell Peppers with Quinoa, Spinach, and Feta Cheese

INGREDIENTS

- 4 huge bell peppers, any color.
- 1 cup cooked quinoa.
- 2 cups fresh spinach, chopped.
- 1/2 cup crumbled feta cheese.
- 1/2 onion, finely chopped
- 2 garlic cloves, minced
- 2 tablespoons olive oil.
- 1 teaspoon of dried oregano or basil.
- Salt and pepper (optional; to taste)
- Fresh parsley (optional for garnish).

INSTRUCTIONS

- Prepare the bell peppers.
- Preheat the oven to 375°F (190° C).
- Slice off the tops of the bell peppers and remove the seeds and membranes.
- Lightly sprinkle olive oil into each pepper and lay upright in a baking dish.
- In a medium skillet, heat 1 tablespoon olive oil. Sauté the chopped onion until transparent, about 3-4 minutes.
- Add the minced garlic and simmer for another 1-2 minutes, or until fragrant.

- Add the chopped spinach and simmer for about 2-3 minutes, or until wilted.

- In a large mixing bowl, mix together the cooked quinoa, sautéed spinach combination, crumbled feta cheese, dried oregano, and a touch of salt and pepper.

- Pack the quinoa and spinach filling snugly into each bell pepper, leaving a little mound on top.

- Bake the stuffed peppers.

- Cover the baking dish with aluminum foil and bake for 25-30 minutes.

- Remove the foil and bake for another 10-15 minutes, or until the peppers are soft and gently brown on top.

- If preferred, garnish the stuffed bell peppers with fresh parsley before serving warm.

Tips:

Choose red, yellow, or orange bell peppers, which are milder and sweeter than green ones.

If your stomach can handle it, add a squeeze of lemon juice to the filling for added brightness.

To make the dish easier on your stomach, avoid using hot items or sauces.

6. Simple Beef and Vegetable Stew with Soft Potatoes and Carrots

INGREDIENTS

- 1 pound of lean beef stew meat, chopped into bite-sized pieces.

- 2 tablespoons olive oil.

- 1 onion, finely chopped

- 2 garlic cloves, minced

- 3 medium carrots, peeled and cut into rounds.

- Two medium potatoes, peeled and chopped

- 2 celery stalks sliced (optional)

- Add 4 cups of low-sodium beef broth and 1 teaspoon of dried thyme or rosemary.

- One bay leaf.

- Salt and pepper (optional; to taste)

- Fresh parsley (optional for garnish).

INSTRUCTIONS

- In a large pot or Dutch oven, heat 1 tablespoon olive oil on medium-high.

- Place the beef stew meat in a single layer and sear on all sides until browned, about 5-7 minutes. Remove the beef and set aside.

- Add the final tablespoon of olive oil to the pot. Sauté the chopped onion and minced garlic for 3-4 minutes, until the onion is transparent.

- Mix in the sliced carrots, diced potatoes, and chopped celery (if using). Cook for an additional 5 minutes, stirring occasionally.

- Return the seared beef to the pot. Combine the low-sodium beef broth, dried thyme, and bay leaf.

- Stir well to mix the ingredients, then bring the stew to a gentle boil.

- Reduce the heat to low, cover, and cook for 45-60 minutes, or until the beef is cooked and the veggies have softened.

- Remove the bay leaf and season the stew with salt and pepper, if preferred.

- Serve the beef and vegetable stew warm, topped with fresh parsley if desired.

Tips:

To make a thicker stew, crush a few chunks of potato in the saucepan to release starch.

To make the food easier on your stomach, avoid using spicy seasonings or hot spices.

This stew can be prepared ahead of time and reheated, as the flavors often develop and improve the following day.

7. Grilled Shrimp with Mashed Butternut Squash and Green Peas

INGREDIENTS

For Grilled Shrimp

- 1 pound of big shrimp, peeled and deveined.

- 2 tablespoons olive oil.

- 1 teaspoon dry herbs (such thyme or oregano)

- Salt and pepper (optional; to taste)

For the mashed butternut squash

- 1 medium butternut squash, peeled and diced

- 2 tablespoons of unsweetened almond milk or low-fat milk.

- 1 tablespoon of olive oil or butter.

- Salt and pepper (optional; to taste)

For the green peas

- 1 cup of frozen green peas.

- 1 tablespoon of olive oil.

- Salt (optional; to taste)

INSTRUCTIONS

- Bring a large pot of water to a boil, then add the cubed butternut squash.
- Cook for 15-20 minutes, or until the squash is soft and easy to penetrate with a fork.
- Drain the squash and transfer to a bowl. Add the olive oil or butter and milk, and mash until smooth. Season with salt and pepper as desired.
- In a bowl, combine the shrimp, olive oil, dry herbs, salt, and pepper.

- Preheat the grill pan or skillet to medium-high heat.
- Grill the shrimp for 2-3 minutes on each side, or until they are pink and cooked through.
- Bring a small pot of water to a boil, then add the frozen green peas.
- Cook for about 3-5 minutes, until soft, then drain and drizzle with olive oil. Season with salt if desired.
- Serve the grilled shrimp with a big scoop of mashed butternut squash and a side of green peas.

Tips:

To make the meal easier on the stomach, avoid using spicy ingredients on the shrimp.

If your stomach tolerates citrus, add a squeeze of fresh lemon juice to the shrimp for an added flavor boost.

If you like, you can use sweet potatoes instead of butternut squash.

8. Vegetable Risotto with Mushrooms, Spinach, and Parmesan Cheese

<u>INGREDIENTS</u>

- 1 cup arborio rice.
- 2 tablespoons olive oil.
- 1 small, finely chopped onion
- 2 garlic cloves, minced
- 1 cup sliced mushrooms (button or cremini)
- 4 cups low-sodium vegetable broth, warmed
- 2 cups fresh spinach.
- 1/2 cup of grated Parmesan cheese.
- Salt and pepper (optional; to taste)

- Fresh parsley (optional for garnish).

<u>INSTRUCTIONS</u>

- Heat the olive oil in a big skillet or pot over medium heat. Sauté the chopped onion for 3-4 minutes, until transparent.
- Cook for an additional 5-7 minutes, or until the mushrooms are soft.
- Add the Arborio rice and simmer for 1-2 minutes, stirring regularly to lightly toast it.
- Add the warmed vegetable broth to the rice, one ladle at a time. Stir continually until the liquid is absorbed before adding the next ladle of broth. Repeat the process until the rice is creamy and fully cooked, which should take around 18-20 minutes.
- Once the rice is cooked and creamy, add the fresh spinach and heat for 1-2 minutes until wilted.
- Remove from heat and add the grated Parmesan cheese. Season with salt and pepper as desired.
- Serve the vegetable risotto warm, topped with fresh parsley if preferred.

Tips:

To make the food stomach-friendly, avoid using spicy ingredients.

To add extra richness, whisk in a little quantity of unsweetened almond milk or low-fat cream at the end.

Depending on your preferences and tolerance, you can add other soft veggies such diced zucchini or bell peppers.

9. Lentil and Vegetable Shepherd's Pie with Mashed Potato Topping

INGREDIENTS

For filling:

- 1 cup dried green or brown lentils, rinsed.
- 2 tablespoons olive oil.
- To prepare, finely chop one onion and mince two garlic cloves.
- Two medium carrots, diced.
- 1 cup of chopped zucchini.
- 1 cup frozen peas.
- 2 cups low-sodium vegetable broth.
- 1 teaspoon of dried thyme or rosemary.
- Salt and pepper (optional; to taste)

For the mashed potato topping:

- 4 medium potatoes, peeled and diced
- 1/2 cup of unsweetened almond or low-fat milk
- 2 tablespoons olive oil or butter.
- Salt and pepper (optional; to taste)

INSTRUCTIONS

- Bring a big pot of water to a boil, then add the cubed potatoes.
- Cook for 15-20 minutes, until the potatoes are cooked.
- Drain the potatoes, then mash them with olive oil or butter and milk until smooth—season with salt and pepper as desired. Set aside.
- In a large skillet, heat the olive oil over medium heat. Sauté the chopped onion for 3-4 minutes, until transparent.
- Combine the minced garlic, diced carrots, and zucchini. Cook for 5-7 minutes, until the vegetables begin to soften.

- Place the rinsed lentils, dried thyme, and vegetable broth in the skillet. Stir thoroughly to mix.
- Bring to a gentle simmer for 25-30 minutes, or until the lentils are cooked. Stir in the frozen peas in the last 5 minutes of cooking.
- Season with salt and pepper as desired.
- Preheat the oven to 375°F (190° C).
- Transfer the lentil and veggie contents to a large baking dish and distribute evenly.
- Spoon the mashed potatoes over the filling and spread evenly with a spatula to cover the whole surface.
- Bake for 20-25 minutes, or until the top is gently browned and the filling bubbles.
- Allow the shepherd's pie to cool for a few minutes before serving.

Tips:

Use white or yellow potatoes to create a creamy, silky topping that is easy to stomach.

To make the food stomach-friendly, avoid using spicy ingredients.

You can add other soft vegetables, like as spinach or bell peppers, if you want.

10. Baked Eggplant Parmesan (Lightly Breaded) with a Side Salad

INGREDIENTS

For the eggplant parmesan:

- 1 large eggplant, cut into 1/4-inch rounds.
- 1 cup of whole wheat breadcrumbs.
- 1/2 cup of grated Parmesan cheese.
- Two giant eggs, beaten
- 1 cup of low-sodium marinara sauce

- 1 cup shredded mozzarella cheese.

- 1 teaspoon of dried oregano or basil.

- Salt and pepper (optional; to taste)

- Olive oil spray or two teaspoons olive oil.

For the side salad:

- 4 cups mixed greens (spinach, arugula or lettuce)

- 1/2 cucumber, sliced.

- 1/2 cup cherry tomatoes (halved)

- 1/4 cup shredded carrots.

- 2 tablespoons olive oil.

- 1 tablespoon balsamic vinegar or lemon juice (optional, but well tolerated)

- Salt and pepper (optional; to taste)

<u>INSTRUCTIONS</u>

- Preheat the oven to 400 °F (200 °C).

- Line a baking sheet with parchment paper, then lightly spray or brush with olive oil.

- Sprinkle salt over the eggplant slices and let them sit for 15-20 minutes to remove extra moisture. Dry them with a paper towel.

- Create a breading station with one bowl of beaten eggs and another bowl of whole wheat breadcrumbs seasoned with Parmesan cheese, dried oregano, salt, and pepper.

- Dip each eggplant slice into the beaten eggs, then coat with the breadcrumb mixture, pressing slightly to ensure even coverage.

- Place the breaded eggplant slices on the prepared baking sheet.

- Lightly spray or pour olive oil on top of the eggplant slices.

- Bake for 20 minutes, flipping halfway through, until the eggplant turns golden and crispy.

- Remove the baking sheet from the oven and spread some marinara sauce on each eggplant slice.
- Sprinkle shredded mozzarella cheese over the marinara sauce.
- Return to the oven and cook for another 10-15 minutes until the cheese is melted and bubbling.
- In a large salad bowl, mix the mixed greens, cucumber slices, cherry tomatoes, and grated carrots.
- Drizzle with olive oil, balsamic vinegar, or lemon juice. Toss lightly to mix, then season with salt and pepper.
- Serve the baked eggplant Parmesan with a fresh side salad for a balanced, ulcer-friendly dinner.

Tips:

To make the dish more digestible, avoid using spicy marinara sauce.

If whole wheat breadcrumbs are too coarse, substitute ordinary breadcrumbs for a softer texture.

You can change the salad ingredients to suit your taste and tolerance and use mild, non-acidic dressings to prevent irritation.

20 Snack and Dessert Recipes

Snacks

- ❖ Banana and Almond Butter Rice Cakes
- ❖ Oatmeal Energy Bites with Honey and Coconut
- ❖ Plain Greek Yogurt with Blueberries and Honey
- ❖ Cucumber and Hummus Slices
- ❖ Apple Slices with Peanut Butter (avoid if acidic fruits trigger symptoms)
- ❖ Soft-boiled egg with Whole Wheat Crackers
- ❖ Smoothie Bowl with Banana, Spinach, and Almond Milk

❖ Baked Sweet Potato Fries with Olive Oil

❖ Avocado Spread on Whole Wheat Toast

❖ Cottage Cheese with Soft Peaches or Pears

Desserts

❖ Banana Oat Cookies (made with mashed bananas and oats)

❖ Rice Pudding with Cinnamon and Honey

❖ Baked Apples with Cinnamon and Raisins

❖ Homemade Applesauce with a Dash of Nutmeg

❖ Chia Seed Pudding with Almond Milk and Berries

❖ Vanilla Yogurt Parfait with Soft Mango and Granola

❖ Peach Smoothie with Yogurt and Honey

❖ Blueberry Muffins (made with whole wheat flour and low sugar)

❖ Banana Ice Cream (blended frozen bananas)

❖ Oat and Banana Pancakes with a Drizzle of Maple Syrup

Low-Acidity Beverages

1. Herbal Teas

Chamomile Tea: Soothes the digestive tract and reduces inflammation.

Ginger Tea: Helps with digestion and reduces nausea.

Peppermint Tea (in moderation): Can soothe the stomach, but avoid if you have acid reflux.

Fennel Tea: Eases bloating and improves digestion.

2. Non-Citrus Smoothies

Banana and Almond Milk Smoothie: Made with banana, almond milk, and a touch of honey.

Oat Milk and Blueberry Smoothie: This gentle, nutritious option is made with oat milk, blueberries, and spinach.

3. Milk Alternatives

Almond Milk: Low in acidity and easy on the stomach.

Oat Milk: Creamy and gentle, suitable for sensitive stomachs.

Coconut Milk (unsweetened): Soothing and low-acid.

4. Low-Acid Juices

Aloe Vera Juice: Known for its soothing properties and helps reduce stomach irritation.

Cabbage Juice: A natural remedy for ulcers, though its taste may need getting used to.

5. Water-Based Options

Coconut Water: Naturally hydrating and low in acidity.

Infused Water: Water infused with cucumber or fresh mint for a refreshing, low-acid drink.

Warm Water with Honey: Soothing and gentle on the stomach.

6. Non-Caffeinated Options

Rooibos Tea: Naturally caffeine-free and low in tannins, making it a tremendous low-acid choice.

Barley Tea: A mild, non-caffeinated beverage that's gentle on the stomach.

CONCLUSION

Healing from a stomach ulcer is a journey that involves time, deliberate choices, and a dedication to supporting your body in ways that promote long-term health.

Throughout this course, we've looked at the significant relationship between what we eat, how we live, and the health of our digestive systems. From understanding the underlying causes of ulcers to implementing a diet rich in healing foods and gentle cooking practices, you've learned to take control of your gut health.

Remember, this journey is about more than just following a set of rules or eliminating foods; it's about learning what works best for your specific body and recovering the joy of eating without pain or suffering.

The recipes, lifestyle recommendations, and natural treatments in this book are intended to empower you—to equip you with a toolkit you can customize to meet your needs and tastes.

It is about developing a new way of eating that cures and provides fulfillment and joy with each meal.

When given the correct tools, your body can heal, and making tiny, regular changes can help lay the stage for recovery.

Celebrate your progress, no matter how modest it may appear. Accept the nourishing power of food, appreciate the support of loved ones, and view each day as an opportunity to go closer to vibrant health.

As you move on, remember that you are not alone. Many people have walked this route before you, discovering comfort, healing, and a new connection with food and their bodies.

With the help of this book and your newfound understanding, you'll have all you need to go on this adventure confidently.

Remember that healing is a continuous process of caring for and loving your body. Trust the process, pay attention to your body's requirements, and enjoy the trip toward a healthier, happy stomach. May this guide be a reassuring companion on your journey to recovery, inspiring you to live a vibrant life free of the pain of stomach ulcers?

Your healing journey begins here, and each step brings you closer to a healthier, brighter, ulcer-free future.